IT'S NOT THE FREAKING WHEAT AMERICA!

I0438203

~ It's Not The Freaking Wheat America ~

It's Not The Freaking Wheat America!

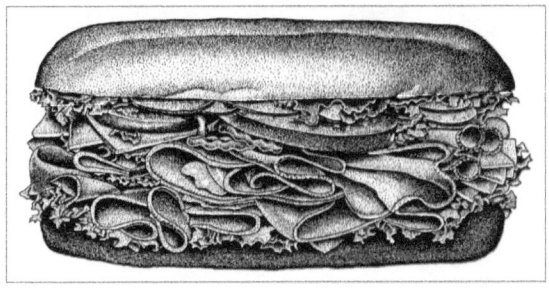

All Illustrations Incuded in this publication were sourced from WWW.SXC.HU and WWW.FREEDIGITALPHOTOS.NET[1]

The Author would like to extent their thanks especially to 'tungphoto' at WWW.FREEDIGITALPHOTOS.NET for the provision of the cover image.

Where possible, all artists will be credited in footnote form beneath each illustration to follow. As with the above Image provided by Billy Alexander

---

1   Image courtesy of Billy Alexander aka ba1969   at WWW.SXC.HU

~ It's Not The Freaking Wheat America ~

COPYRIGHT

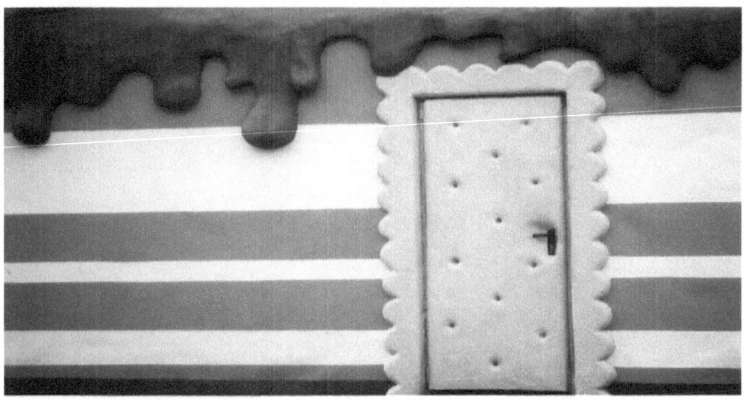

---

2 Image courtesy of Loredana Bejerita aka l-o-l-a at www.sxc.hu

~ It's Not The Freaking Wheat America ~

Contents

INTRODUCTION

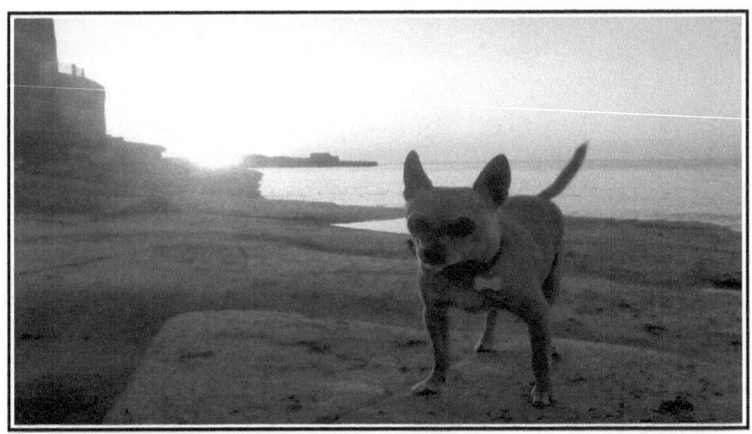

Hi America, my name is Chelsea, and despite the surname that you might have noted as you moved to inspect this books details, I'm afraid that I'm in no way related to Chelsea Manning of Wikileaks infamy.

I have however, written this book in order to put a spotlight on the real reason why America has an exponentially increasing weight problem at present. One which rather than jump on the bread and carbohydrates are pure evil bandwagon, is going to tell you in the simplest of terms possible, why you are struggling with your weight right now, and what you can legitimately do about that.

1

I have a one size fits all solution to long term sustainable weight loss, and I really want to share that with you.

What I don't have however, is a quick fix for anyone. I lost 100 pounds but it took me three years. Don't therefore pay for and dive into this, if you're desperate for a quick fix for how you presently feel about yourself.

That said, I spent half my life dieting and trying all kinds of ways to loose weight, and you know what? Yeah most of them worked, but those that did only worked in the short term.

What I'm therefore going to do here, is take you through what is really making it hard for you to stay in shape in the first place, and then say okay, take it or leave it, here's the solution.

Of course, whether you take my advice or not is entirely up to you. In the very least case though, I hope that I can at least put a bug in your ear.
Enjoy.

(By the way the above picture is of my dog Art. He'll feature briefly in my story later).

Believing What We Need To

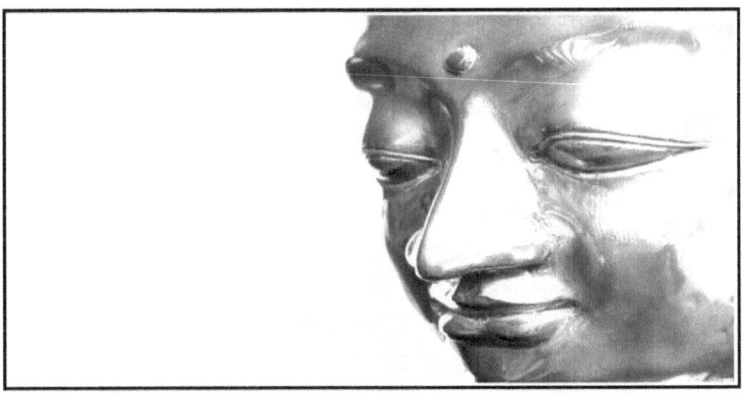

"I mean look at me," my friend Robyn says as we pull out of Applebee's. "I'm in the best shape I've been in my entire life, I've got a great job and I've got a great man in my life."[3]

Her eyes catch mine in the rear view mirror as if to make sure that I agree. Reflexively then, I reach for a cigarette. Its true what they say, they really are a social crutch.

"I can't believe you're still smoking those," she says lowering the passenger side window further than is comfortable for me to smoke out of.

---

3   Image courtesy of Rick Tolboom aka ricky01 at www.sxc.hu

I want to say, "well Robyn, I can't believe how much you just ate." But that would be cruel.

You see, Robyn's not in great shape. Like nearly 34% of Americans she's hideously obese. She confided in me once that her size had all but destroyed her sex life, and despite her present enthusiasm, I can't imagine that that issue has been resolved.

In fact, in the three years since I last saw her, Robyn's got so big that I couldn't even put my arms around her in the airport arrival lounge.

Out of the window as we head down Mills Avenue, we pass a pediatrics, a Florida Heart group center, a center for radiology and a center for digestive health.

Nearly all of these places however, are neighbored by, or just a stones throw away from yet another sandwich bar, pizzeria, or hot dog parlor. And I realize why Robyn, will despite all her best efforts, likely only ever get bigger.

You see, the problem isn't that Robyn's obese. The problem is that America is obese. Every mile we drive, we're surrounded by Chick-fil-A, Denny's and master of them all, McDonald's drive throughs.

Likewise, it's impossible to find a retail park which

doesn't have the parking lot surrounded by even more, all be them usually niche fast food franchises. And whilst the heart and soul of American culture has always been inalienable from the American family dinner table, the economic boom and bust years of the twenty first century, have given rise to what I like to call America's Cheese Cake Factory culture.

It's simply not the norm if you like, for most of us to squash around Brady Bunch, or even Malcolm In The Middle stylized family dinner tables any more.

Rather, we're either all too busy to eat together, or it's simply cheaper and easier for us to outsource the preparation of the majority of our snacks and meals each day, to the pseudo glamorous giants of American corporatism.

In fact, most of us are so used to eating either alone or with strangers, that when we are forced to gather and eat as families like we used to, we feel awkward and uncomfortable.

Moreover, just like my friend Robyn, America as a nation seems to be in absolute denial of the fact, that it as a country and a culture has a food problem.

Where Robyn blames her big bones, her under active thyroid, and even other people for using the gym when she'd like to, America blames its modern day citizens demand for and need of convenience.

Personal choice is apparently to blame for America's obesity pandemic, and appropriation of blame for the sake of economic prosperity, must never it seems, be laid at the door of America's food industry.

This being the case, American culture is perpetually inundated with diet books and get fit quick guides, all of which blame specific food groups for making people overweight.

Some say that cutting out wheat is the answer to a flatter stomach and healthier digestion. Some others advocate vegetarianism. And many others over the past decade especially, have insisted that high protein diets, with sever restrictions on any kind of carbohydrate intake, is the way to go for a healthier and younger looking you.

What few ever allude to however, is the fast food human mouse trap slotted under every office workers desk, and every city commuters driving seat. The one thats lunch breaks spent surrounded by the noise and intoxicating aroma of at least a dozen take out outlets.

Further, although each such publication has its merits, what Americans tend to do these days, is pick and read diet books which they perceive as being geared towards telling them what they want to believe in the first place.

My friend Robyn for instance, is a meatloaf and burger nut. As such, rather than find a diet book on her coffee table detailing the virtues of vegetarianism, there's presently one emblazoned with a picture of a large ham steaming angelically beneath a golden halo.

My sister on the other hand, prefers to believe that calorie counting, and eating only alkaline forming foods, is the one and only way to stay trim and limber.

This being the case, diet books usually found resting on the side of my sisters sofa, are ones which praise the merits of juicing, whilst steering clear of any kind of bread, cereal or pasta.

Cumulatively in fact, America's literary love affair with by and large always at odds diet and nutrition manuals, can itself be argued to have added to America's obesity problem.

You see, there isn't any middle ground anywhere. No single book seems to want to address the fact that it's America's relationship with food overall which needs to change, not just the nations relationship with bread and red meat.

Moreover, adherence to one nutritional doctrine over another, often sees people crash dieting. My friend Robyn did the Atkins diet in 2004 and lost twenty pounds. When however, her metabolism adjusted to her new regimen and she started to regain weight, she panicked and for all intensive purposes tried to starve herself through juicing.

Wouldn't it be nice therefore, if someone could come along, sit you down, and really tell you how to loose weight? Maybe even tell you why you presently struggle with your size, and give you a few solid tips on how to fix that?

Here it is though, this book is not going to make you thin, happy or beautiful. Only you can do these things.

In fact, as a guy in a bar in Middle River once told me, anyone anywhere is only ever five minutes away from the rest of their life, and what's running through anyone's mind in that five minutes, isn't anyone's business but their own.

If you want to loose weight, yeah, I'll tell you how you can do it. If you want to look and feel better about yourself, I can even tell you how to start working towards that too.

There isn't any such thing however, as ten steps to a brand new beautiful you. All there is is you, and a decision which you have or haven't made yet to start bettering yourself, for yourself in the long term.

8

I mean sure, you can try drinking multicolored fruit smoothies and vegetable juice for ten or twelve days, and sure you'll likely feel fantastic. But hey, here's the kicker kids, do you really think that there would be that many crash diet books on the market if any of them actually worked?

Instead, what I'm going to give you is a long term, balanced solution to better health. I'm going to tell you to stop wasting money on supplements and diet pills, and I'm going to ask you to simply start taking responsibility for your own body and your own life.

Moreover, I'm not going to target this book at the organic lime juice guzzling, "it has to be true because it's written by a world famous nutritionist" crowd.

I'm not a world famous nutritionist. Nor a world famous anything else for that matter.

More importantly, I'm not going to try and use this book to sell anyone the idea at they could be the next Cameron Diaz.

You see, in many respects the idea that being thin equates to being beautiful, is part of the reason that America is presently in the mess that it's in.

Being thin doesn't equal being beautiful any more

than being beautiful makes anyone a better and more loved individual, or being fabulously wealthy equals happiness.

Moreover, what putting that idea in someone's head does, is make them reach for the cookie dough when they realize that they can't fit into their favorite shirt or dress any more.

It makes people call off dates at the last minute because they don't think that they will stand a chance with the person they are about to have dinner with. And worst of all, it makes people who do get in shape, even more susceptible to binge eating, the development of eating disorders, and even complete relapses into states of chronic obesity.

I mean what do you do when you've been told for all of your adult life that happiness is dependent on what you eat and how many times a week you work out, only to finally get there and realize that everyone your working out with is actually really superficial?

In fact, although this book will by no stretch of anyone's imagination be a dating guide, it might even go so far to advise you how to finally find your ideal other half.

You see, being single and overweight in America is a bit of a sick joke. On one side of the street you've got a big girl who thinks that she'll only ever find happiness when she's at least got herself down to a size sixteen. And on the other side of the street you've often got a big guy who thinks he'll never find a girl because of his own waist size.

Sometimes then I wish I could be like Dr Oz or Oprah, and be granted some divine right to barge into such peoples lives and say, "okay Phil, you're a big guy who likes your fried chicken, but is always feeling down on his luck because of his weight. Well guess what? See Sarah over there? She feels exactly the same most days, and as well as loving fried chicken, she'd just love for someone to notice her just as much as you would."

You see, whilst so many of us are striving blindly for unattainable physical perfection, we somehow seem to blinker ourselves to the fact that there's over two hundred and fifteen million people in America in any one moment, who are all essentially in the same boat as we are.

Of course, I'm not saying that it's fine to be as big as you might be. It's not. And at the back of your mind if you are overweight, there's likely a depressive catalog already, of every one of the possible health implications of every extra pound you're presently carrying.

What I am saying though, is that everyone seems to think that they have to face their weight alone

11

when really this just makes things harder for a lot of people.

Therefore if you are one of these people who thinks that they want to loose weight just so that they can more comfortably meet people, the last thing you need is another diet book. Instead, do yourself a real favor, and get a gym buddy.

As for me, I'm not overly pretty, rich, or anywhere near as toned as any celebrity you might want to being to mind. I am happy though.

Moreover, although I haven't created any kind of miraculous dietary or exercise regimen which I wish to gift to the world, I, unlike many people reading this, sincerely don't worry about developing many of the diseases you do, or having to watch my weight bounce up and down like the Richter scale.

I'm simply me. A healthy, balanced American woman in her thirties, who wants to take the opportunity to say "hey America, can I talk to you for a moment?"

Because you know what? As much as I love being sat next to my friend Robyn as we turn into her new apartment garage, I'm tired of watching her and America just get bigger every time I see them.

IF AMERICA WAS AN ELEPHANT

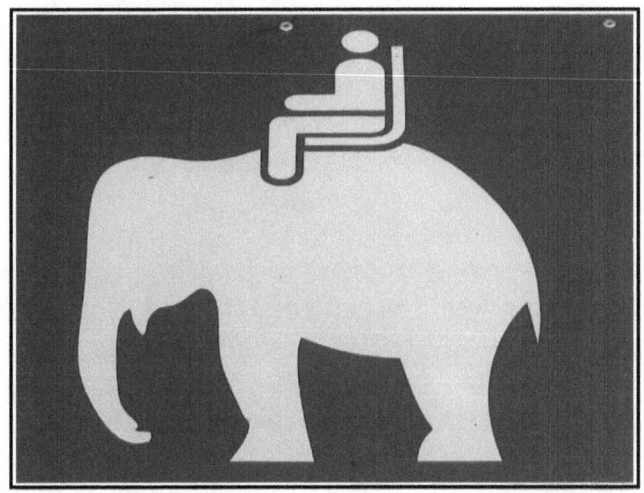

It's 7am. The phone which you put on charge last night by your bedside starts to vibrate sound alarm. You check your messages whilst changing yesterdays filter in the coffee machine. [4]

In the den, MTV starts shouting something at you from Nicki Minaj, and a following commercial break stretches for nearly the full five minutes it takes you to chew through a bowl of cereal and sip your coffee.

---

4   IMAGE COURTESY OF CLODIA PORTEOUS   AKA PORCN001   AT WWW.SXC.HU

You shower, pocket your phone and snatch your car keys. Outside the sky is the same soup spill of gray as it was yesterday, and so you're actually looking forward to getting to work and getting what time you need to spend outdoors over with already.

The year is 2014, and for all intensive purposes this is your life. You will come home later, throw something in the microwave and switch on the television.

Then, you'll spend the rest of the time that's yours, flicking your eyes between it and your tablet computer, as you broadcast via wifi, your views on the book you started reading today and what you think of Miley Cyrus' new music video.

Of course, the above narrative changes somewhat when you add children into the equation. However, for the sake of argument, if you could somehow superimpose this scene over an average American morning from the 1980's, very little would jump out as different.

Sure, instead of the messages on your cell phone, you'd likely see yourself sorting through the mail. However, aside from our touch screens and what's on MTV, very little in America has visibly changed in the last twenty or so years.

Under societies overall surface however, something

14

has changed.

Because of our increasing waistlines and a host of other reasons which are never really elaborated upon, we're constantly being told that one in every three of us will likely experience cancer in our lifetimes.

Similarly, Internet banner adds routinely suggest that just as many of us should expect to experience early on set dementia and diabetes. Whilst even our TV's and radios have recently taken to telling us that 1 in 88 of American children in 2014, will likely now register as Autistic.

America if you like, is sick. Further, and although no one seems to want to talk about it, America seems to be getting even sicker with every passing year.

Whereas in 2000, 1 in 150 American children would register as autistic, the fourteen years since have seen instances of autism almost double.

Likewise, whereas in 2001, 20.4 million American's were suffering from asthma, in just thirteen years this number has increased by almost a full quarter to 24.6 million.

Indeed, as well as allergies, digestive disorders, depression and a host of other medical conditions, obesity in America has itself more than doubled in prevalence, since just 1995.

What I find particularly troubling about such trends however, is that whereas animal populations seen to suffer marked declines in their general health and well being, will in most cases have such declines attributed to changes in their immediate environment; any decline in human health is put strictly down to patient specific stimulus.

Cancer will first and foremost be attributed to the diet and smoking status of the person suffering the disease. Then, if alcohol, sunlight exposure and/or unprotected sexual intercourse can't be attributed with having spurred its on set, an inherent genetic fault will be blamed.

Further, although rapidly becoming common place conditions such as Autism have no officially recognized cause, any suggestion that the condition might be attributable (even in part) to diet or childhood vaccination programs, is considered scientific heresy.

This despite the fact that independent studies now routinely show obvious parallels between historical vaccination programs and initial diagnosis's of the condition.

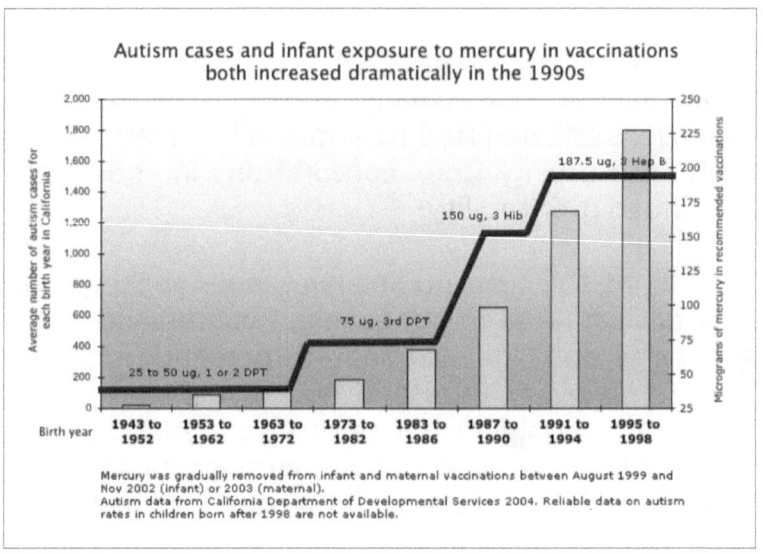

In fact, although America's political and scientific community seem able to readily accept that PCB chemicals used in American industry between the 1930's and 1970's, are still effecting the health of polar bears in the Arctic. The minute that anyone draws attention to the fact that America's since 1995 explosion in obesity, correlates directly to things like America's since the same time cultivation and consumption of genetically modified food products; the doors of America's scientific and political hierarchy swing firmly closed.

America it seems, simply can't ever bring itself to question the actions of what essentially is its ruling corporate elite.

17

Should evidence ever surface which suggests that some kind of corporate produced common consumable might actually be bad for people, such assertions are nullified by armies of lawyers tasked with preserving the corporation in questions continued profitability.

This being the case, no one ever looks at things like why autism rates in Venezuela, (where children by and large don't get vaccinated) presently stand at just 1.1 in every thousand. Whilst autism rates in America not only increase every year, but can even be seen to increase in parallel with increases in the amount of mercury used in American vaccines.

However, before this gets too political, lets just take a look back at our average American morning where you get out of bed and eat your cereal etc.

You see, although it looks and tastes the same as it did in the 1980's, breakfast cereal in America is for the most part now inclusive of a plethora of genetically modified organisms which didn't even exist twenty years ago.

Similarly, because genetically modified crops require heavy spraying with glyphosate, there are even traces of pesticides in America's cereal.

Indeed, (and as if that wasn't enough) the milk which you put on that cereal contains artificial growth hormones which only came into use in 1993, and which are actually banned in the United Kingdom, Europe and Canada.

Moving away from just our food for a moment though, it is also the case that the majority of American urban areas, are now blanketed by electromagnetic radiation.

Wifi, 3 and 4G telecommunications systems, smart meters, and even home and office based cordless phone base stations, are after all, now constantly transmitting and receiving microwave radiation all around us. Radiation which is strong enough to pass through several layers of solid stonework, and radiation which telecommunications firms themselves are well aware can cause cancer and even inheritable genetic abnormalities.

"When human blood cells are irradiated with electromagnetic fields, clear damage to hereditary material has been demonstrated and there have been indications of an increased cancer risk."

The above for example, was included in a 2003 international patent submission from Swisscom AG, a major telecommunications provider in Switzerland, in regard to technology which it then wished to patent in order to negate the physiological effects of Swisscom products.

So here it is. Although for the most part everything still looks the same as it did in the 80's, you didn't just get out of bed and eat your cereal this morning.

Rather, you woke from your sleep in a 3G and quite possibly wifi saturated room, you proceeded to devour a bowl of genetically modified grains coated in glyphosate and bovine growth hormones, and as soon as you went outside, you entered a constant pulsing haze of electricity. One which immediately began interfering with your mood, metabolism and endocrine system.

Of course, I could mention a plethora of other products and subsequent human habitat changes however, I'm really trying hard to keep this simple.

In fact, to simplify even better, try to imagine that the whole world is a zoo, and that every country in that zoo is represented by a single animal exhibited in a single enclosure.

To simplify even further in fact, lets make every animal an elephant of the exact same age, with a perfect previous health record.

Also lets say that a week spent in this zoo, is the equivalent of a whole year here in the real world.

Now, lets imagine that one day America's zoo keeper is approached by a business man who says "hey, do you realize that you could save thousands of dollars every year, simply by feeding America some cool new genetically modified food?"

The business man then says that he could even put a wifi hot spot by America's enclosure, and in doing so attract more visitors than there are to all the other elephants in the park.

Since the proposition sounds great, America's keeper signs on the dotted line and for a little while everything is fantastic.

Twenty weeks later however, America has put on 30% extra weight, she's lethargic all the time, has a host of gastric complaints, and is even showing signs of clinical depression.

This being the case, both the zoo's owner and a vet come to visit, and the first thing that they ask, (just like veterinarians and family Md's around the world usually do) is, "okay, have you changed America's diet in any way recently?"

Moreover, as soon as its been established that America isn't actually eating what the other elephants are eating, the first thing that any MD is likely to suggest, is that she's put back on her old diet, (at least temporarily) to see if there is any improvement.

In the real world however, Americans by and large aren't even allowed to make that decision for

21

themselves. You see, apparently, even so much as labeling GMO products would be too much for the people who produce them.

Make no mistake however, I'm not going to spend from here on in trying to convince you that you should start making an effort to avoid GMO and go cable rather than wireless.

You see, the thing about us American's is that we're stubborn as mules. In fact, as Mark Twain once said, 'It's easier to fool people than to convince them that they have been fooled.'

It is perhaps worth keeping in mind however, that due simply to the amount of money spent lobbying governments all around the world by Big Tobacco, smoking wasn't ever officially declared bad for people either.

In fact, it wasn't until the industry insider Jeffrey Wigand, appeared on CBS's 60 minutes program in 1996, that nicotine itself was even admitted to being addictive.

All I am trying to do here then, is point out a simple and verifiable fact. This being that in tandem with America's health and obesity crisis, the food produce that's on your average Americans weekly grocery list has itself changed exponentially.

What anyone wants to do with that fact is entirely

up to them.

For me personally, I was a hundred pounds overweight, I had irritable bowel syndrome, I was taking Alprazolam every morning, and I thought when I first thought about this, "okay what's to loose by just cutting this stuff out for a while?" And that's how it's got to be for everyone.

Moreover, it ain't easy. Most people are aware for example, that most of America's corn is genetically modified. However, what most people don't realize, is that fructose derived from corn is a staple ingredient in everything from your kids breakfast cereal, to your soda and your chewing gum.

In fact, the 'modified starch' in your favorite sliced cold meats is largely derived from corn kernels, and everything from the adhesive on envelopes, to the sorbitol in any toothpaste you might use, is rendered from it.

Getting this stuff out of your body completely, isn't therefore just about you being willing to alter your and perhaps your whole families diet and personal hygiene regimen. It's about you getting your head down and doing some serious research into what's actually in, literally everything which you are putting in or on your body everyday.

Rather however, than be appreciated as too difficult or time consuming, what this does is really rather incredible.

You see, by deciding that you don't want even the smallest trace of something in your diet any more, you start to fundamentally recondition your entire relationship with food.

To demonstrate, I used to shop in Safeway every week and I used to literally shovel packets of sliced ham into my shopping cart. (Being a grilled cheese fanatic, I'd go through a packet or so every two days).

However, when I realized that I couldn't have sliced ham any more because of the modified soy content, I had to either resign myself to never tasting a grilled cheese (with ham) again, or set about finding a solution.

Less than thrilled to say the least, with the prospect of having to face life without this particular vice, I in the end settled on buying a whole joint of ham every week (or two depending on the size) before cooking and slicing it myself. And although this in itself might seem meaningless, this completely changed my emotional relationship with something that until then had been a ready in five minute snack food.

You see, I'm not wealthy, far from it. Therefore selecting a joint in the first place became a mental and physical process in of itself.

I'd appreciate the weight against the price, against how much space I had in the freezer. And then I'd think of whether I even had time this Saturday to roast, slice, and portion up the thing in the first place.

What I soon started to find however, was that it was actually much better value (in most cases) to buy a whole joint. Meanwhile, the quality of what I was tasting and putting through my own digestive system improved exponentially.

More importantly however, what establishing this process quite quickly resulted in, was me divorcing myself psychologically from the idea that preparing a grilled cheese as a snack during a break in Breaking Bad, was in any way convenient.

Further, this was something that came about without me having to forcibly limit myself from the experience of a grilled cheese, like I used to when I used to diet.

What I then noticed, was that by throwing a more substantial slice of ham into my grilled cheese's, I was making them considerably more filling.

Whereas then, my old self would often run back to the kitchen during the next commercial break to quickly prepare another one, this time around I'd actually satisfy my appetite in a single serving.

Furthermore, this is just one example. Because I was making an effort to avoid consuming any kind of GMO product, I had to avoid drinking literally any kind of soda ever again.

This being the case, and after running through the known adverse health effects of additives in even 100% natural fruit juices, I opted for boiling five liters of water on the stove every second day, before throwing in three or so green tea bags and adding the juice of a couple of freshly squeezed lemons.

Usually carrying a refillable water bottle with me anyway, I then simply took to taking my own 'soda' out and about with me. And not only do I not miss that sickly sweet sticky feeling on my teeth, but ever since then I've felt fantastic.

Moreover, once again I fundamentally reconditioned my psychological relationship with something that I was putting into my body everyday, and that's something critical to keep in mind. You see, America's health and obesity problem is just as much about our nations psychological and emotional relationship with food, as it is about what we're actually eating.

WHERE IS YOUR MIND AMERICA?

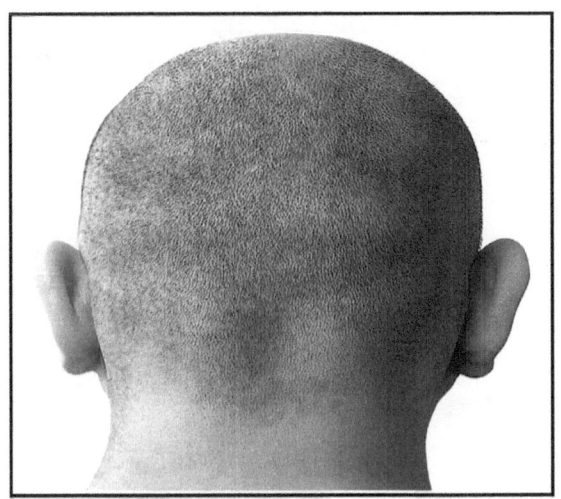

Okay, I know that I probably ruffled a few peoples feathers by diving straight into the whole GMO debate. Here however, is the simple crux of the matter: You and no-one else is responsible for what you put into your body. I'm no more responsible for telling people what they should and shouldn't eat, than whoever is in the White House, or whoever is running the FDA at any one moment. [5]

---

5   IMAGE COURTESY OF CECILIA PICCO AKA CHUX AT WWW.SXC.HU

One of the problems with America at present however, is that people seem to have got it into their heads that it's the American way just to let other people and other institutions decide what they should eat, drink, wear and even talk about.

This being the case, many Americans have effectively outsourced their psychological and emotional relationship with food. And that's something that's a real shame.

Whereas once for instance, we associated satisfying our hunger with cakes and biscuits which we or our extended family members had cooked up over the previous weekend, most of us presently associate satisfying our hunger with a quick trip to Taco Bell.

In fact, let's say that you are in your favorite burger place or pizzeria, and you suddenly decide that you want to know what the actual ingredients are of what it is that you are eating. You see, the person who served you won't be able to tell you. Neither in fact, will the girl or guy in the back who cooked up your meal in the first place.

Rather, the bread base, the meat that made your burger or pizza topping, and even the fries and salady bits that your meal was served with, was all delivered preprepared in the first place.

Of course, many places will boast that they use

only "the freshest and finest ingredients," but hey that's just marketing. The simple fact is that neither you or the person who just prepared your meal, actually knows what you are about to put into your body.

To demonstrate, as recently as January 2014, it was revealed that the sandwich producer Subway, had until that time been adding an industrial chemical called azodicarbonamide, (usually used in shoe rubber) to its sandwich bread.

Indeed, although Subway has since removed this additive, it has since been revealed that over 500 American food products sold under 130 different brand names still contain it.

America as a society, has therefore gone from one in which fifty to sixty years ago, many people would still bake their own bread and therefore know exactly what was in it, to one in which just as many people now sit around unwittingly eating shoe rubber. And this is something which frustrates the hell out of me. Especially when I hear people in my gym class talking about how they have just read this extraordinarily enlightening book, about how wheat itself is to blame for all of America's health woes.

You see, I got news for you America, it's not the freaking wheat that's the problem here. The problem with bread in America, is that most of it is baked using potassium bromate, an FDA approved but banned everywhere else chemical added so as to reduce baking times.

Further, the problem with our wheat based cakes, pasta and pastry goodies, isn't the fact that wheat grass itself has been grossly over cultivated. What you should be more worried about, is the fact that most such produce is made to look pretty via the use of banned outside of America coloring agents derived from coal tar.

There isn't however, any kind of cognitive process any more, in which Americans actually think about what they are eating.

Lets imagine for example, that you're a young boy or girl in 1930's North Dakota, and your mum or one of your grandparents is teaching you how to bake bread. You'd start with some white or wholemeal flour, you'd add some salt yeast and warm milk or water and you would mix and kneed the resulting dough, before leaving it to rise for the afternoon.

Imagine then, how nightmarish it would be for such a tutor of this simple recipe, to see us in the present day adding ceramic elasticity compounds, coal tar sourced colorings, potassium salts, bovine puss and growth hormones, and even genetically modified additives to our dough!

In fact, to demonstrate how intellectually and

emotionally dislocated we have become from our food, just try asking someone if they actually know what's in the burger bun they are about to eat. You see, likely you'll be met with a roll of the eyes and a look of incredulity, before whoever you have asked says something like, "er bread....." like your the one not quite with the program.

Of course, it's not the case that people don't know that they need things like vitamins, minerals, and different types of fats and proteins. America does after all, have a booming health supplement industry.

Rather, people just seem to presently see things like bread, processed meat, half and half, and even foods such as pizza, as stand alone ingredients of meals, not products which themselves are made up of tens, if not hundreds of ingredients themselves.

Moreover, Americans tend to think of food as just fuel for their bodies. Hence why health and fitness magazines, only ever seem to want to talk about how you should cut down on carb's.

Realistically however, what America needs to do is sit down and realize that as well as the main five food groups, it's got a hell of a lot of industrial junk in its diet.

You see, you can't burn off the industrial fire retardant hexabromocyclododecane found in 90%

of American meat, fish and dairy. And whether you like it or not, the BHT, BHA, and TBHQ benzoate preservatives that most Americans eat everyday, can't be shifted no matter how many sessions at the gym you manage to fit in each week.

Instead, and just like with polar bears and PCB's, most non-organic substances that your body doesn't have a clue what to do with, simply get stored in our fat cells.

In fact, you might not actually be overeating at all. However, as soon as your body realizes that it can't actually do anything with the brominated vegetable oil you just guzzled with your last diet soda, it's got no option but to store what it can't break down as fat.

Further, although it is possible to detox, and although our fat cells are good at encapsulating this stuff, these chemicals do slowly leech out over time into our bloodstreams.

The best way to think about this, being to imagine rusty toxic waste drums corroding away at the bottom of the ocean; each one slowly releasing more and more carcinogenic material into our body environments.

Indeed, when you feed mice and rats diets inclusive of equivocal amounts of the chemicals and additives which we eat every day, they usually develop things like cancer, diabetes and gastrointestinal disorders.

For me then, the fact that one in two of all American males should expect to contract some kind of cancer in their lifetimes makes perfect sense. I mean the beer bellies and the backsides which most of them are walking around with, aren't just made up of artery clogging fat cells.

Rather, because of America's love affair with arsenic fed, and MSG infused chicken, deep fried in hydrogenated vegetable oil, the average American male is his own personal toxic waste dump.

Aside however, from the fact that most of the food that your average American eats everyday is riddled with artificial preservatives, colorings and chemical flavor enhancers, (many of which are derived from petroleum) what we further fail to realize is that most of it is nutritionally dead to start with.

Have you ever noticed for example, how a lot of overweight Americans standing in line at Denny's, tend to have hard calluses on their elbows? As well as greasy and reddened skin, and in general skin complaints overall?

You see, both dry and greasy skin, as well as conditions from eczema to acne and psoriasis, are not only much more prevalent in overweight people, but are all also sure signs of long term vitamin and mineral deficiencies.

Essentially in fact, the reason that many Americans are overweight to begin with, is due simply to their bodies actually being starved of any real kind of nourishment. Moreover, how do our bodies tell us when they need something? They tell us that we're hungry!

However, if that hunger is only ever getting satisfied with beige colored junk from a foil bag of chips, a foot long sub, or a grilled cheese, your body likely just isn't getting what it actually needs.

In fact, by satisfying our appetites in such a way, we're actually exasperating the problem by forcing our bodies to waste valuable resources metabolizing nutritionally dead carbohydrates, whilst neutralizing as fat, all the industrial junk tagging along for the ride.

This being the case, and although most people with weight problems are ashamed to ever admit it, most Americans are actually constantly physically hungry.

Hell, I know that I used to be. I'd have breakfast, grab something before work, grab something on my break, already feel like I was ready for dinner by lunch time; and even on my way home I'd grab something from a drive through, before preparing dinner and finishing the evening with a grilled cheese.....or three.

In fact, I'd never dare admit it, but all I thought about for most of the day was food. Every minute was one passing as part of a count down toward my next eating experience.

The kicker then, is that all dieting to loose weight actually does, is exasperate this feeling of being hungry, because we're actually giving our already starving bodies even less food and likely even less nutrition.

Oh sure, we start new diet regimens and we take time out to flap around and tell everyone how amazing it is that we're not hungry any more. But lets face it, how long does that feeling really last? A week? A day? An hour?

Moreover, all diets will tell you to cut something out, whether that's bread, meat, potatoes, or sometimes even solid food completely.

If however, you're a big girl with a chronic dry skin problem and a general feeling of lethargy, juicing or cutting down on the red meat and dairy for any length of time, is actually the worst thing you can do.

You see, chronic dry skin and lethargy are the main signs that someone is deficient in vitamin B12. One that our bodies metabolize optimally when it arrives in the form of eggs, shellfish, and beef and tuna.

Further, although your average Walgreen's is topped full of vitamin and mineral concoctions, promising everything from better eyesight and hair quality, to even increased longevity; the simple fact is that your body is designed to get what it needs from the food you put into it.

In fact, when I'm at work and lets say Nick on the desk over from mine, is munching through processed rice crackers all day under the deranged belief that they have some kind of negative calorie value, and still packed full of nutrients; I feel like screaming.

Truth be told, I want to get up, get hold of him, and scream, "where is your mind America?" I mean come on, you've been eating rice crackers since the 90's and where has it actually got you?

You see, the truth is that America's fatter and uglier and more diseased than ever.

Therefore do yourself a favor and go to the bathroom. Once you're in there open your mouth and have a good look at your teeth. You see, human beings are omnivores. That's why we've got sets of molars for grinding down vegetable matter, and fangs and incisors for ripping apart bits of dead animals.

Now, take off your shirt pants and underwear, breathe out, look at yourself in the mirror, and ask yourself if you think you look healthy. You see, a lot of us don't appreciate how bad the problem with our bodies has actually got.

By and large in fact, we spend our lives hiding ourselves from ourselves, just as much as we do other people.

Now however, take hold of a fold of belly, thigh or even forearm and just look at it.

You see, all your life you've been told that what's in there is the fault of you being to easily seduced by the Colonels secret recipe for fried chicken. You've been told that it's an over cultivated plants fault, and you've been told that your girth might even be attributable to inherent flaws in your own genetic material.

Never however, has anyone simply pointed out the fact that most of what you're eating every day is complete and utter garbage, and that the fat you're carrying is actually there to save the rest of your body from exposure to the worst of it.

Of course, it still needs to go. But here's the thing. For you to realistically start getting rid of all that extra insulation, you're going to have to go into your kitchen and empty it of every single piece of processed food.

This means anything in a tin, and this means anything with an expiry date further than a week away, that's not a loose fruit or vegetable. Likewise, this means any meat or fish that you've got in the freezer that's been seasoned or breaded for you, and any kind of microwave meal.

This means your bread, your milk, any and all candy, and even any salt and stock cubes which you have lying around.

In fact when you're finished, you should only have loose fruit and vegetables, any joints of meat which you already had in the fridge or freezer, and any packets of died fruit or vegetables which you might have had already.

There shouldn't be a single pot of yogurt, a single cookie, a single tub of ice cream, or a single can of soda lurking anywhere.

However, here's the thing. I'm not going to tell you now that you can't ever again eat a burger and fries with lashings of ketchup and mayonnaise. Neither am I going to tell you that you can't ever again have your favorite deserts, pasta dishes or fried chicken.

What I am going to say though, is that if you're serious about taking control of your own weight and in general health, you're going to have to start making everything you like for yourself, from ingredients that you know you can trust.

Yeah it's going to be an uphill journey for a while in the beginning. I mean lets face it, most American's idea of cooking something from scratch these days, is putting a shop bought pie or pizza in the oven.

However, when we cook for ourselves and when we are forced to plan our meals and snacks ahead, we don't just completely rebuild our emotional relationship with the food we're consuming.

Rather we assert intellectual control, over what we decide for and against putting into our bodies in the first place.

In fact, although you will only experience it if you decide to go all the way yourself, after six or so months of preparing from scratch everything that you eat and drink, you can actually taste the chemicals and preservatives in each and every sip of soda or canned soup which you might choose to taste.

Likely in fact, because abstaining from soda for any length of time will lower your bodies tolerance to things like aspartame, drinking a whole bottle will probably give you a headache.

Further, this regimen won't make you drop a jean size or even a dress size before Christmas.

However, once we are eating food full of nutrients and free of artificial chemicals and emulsifiers, our bodies start to nourish themselves from within.

As such you will find that you have more energy. You'll start feeling more awake and assertive, and as soon as that happens, you'll perhaps start thinking about going for a walk around the block, or if you do that already, the next block as well.

You will if you like, start a slow physiological process of reinvigorating your whole body. One that will see you loose weight in the long term, just not overnight.

Of course, there are always going to be people who say that they simply don't have the time. Not to mention many others, who simply can't believe that agencies such as the FDA don't really have their best interests at heart.

In fact, if I actually finish this thing, it's likely to come under fire from foodies around the world rallying in defense of their favourite burger and chicken sandwich joints. (Not to mention the conventional diet book crowd).

You know what though? That's fine.

You see, I'm just telling you what I have done to better myself for myself.

If you don't think you have the time, that's really none of my business. If you don't want to turn over your soda and start googling each individual additive in order to see what their proven health effects are, that's your choice.

But hey, if you think that I'm trying to attack the heart and soul of America by calling out a cartoon clown for feeding you poison, just do yourself a favor and go look in the mirror America.

~ It's Not The Freaking Wheat America ~

UNDERSTANDING HOW YOU GOT HERE

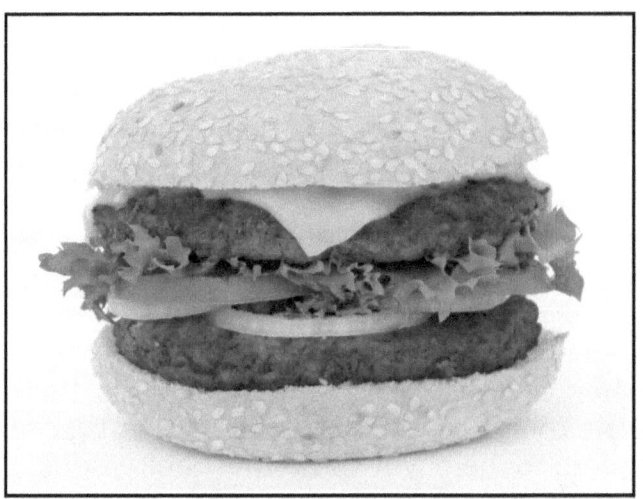

"Wait a minute," you're probably thinking. "Didn't this uppity bitch start this book by saying that she's a smoker? How dare she lecture me on what to eat and how to stay healthy". And you know what? You're right, I am a smoker.[6]

I tried my first cigarette when I was 16 and less than a year later was your typical forty to sixty a day

---

6   IMAGE COURTESY OF ROB OWEN-WAHL 'AN EASTBOURNE WEBSITE DESIGNER' : WWW.DESIGNFISHSTUDIO.COM

chain smoker. In fact, all I was really missing was a trailer and a beer in hand for most hours of the day.

Of course, that's my attempt at a small joke. Make no mistake though, smoking ruins you. It hurts you financially. It ruins your looks. And you don't realize it until you finally do decide to quit, but it really makes you stink.

In fact, smoking is actually a lot like overeating. It gets addictive real fast, and when people start to have a problem cutting back a bit, they push it to the back of their mind and box it up under, 'something else to get around to dealing with one day..... Just not today.'

Further, and just like dieting, there's a thousand and one things presently on the market supposedly designed to help you kick the habit. Books, self hypnosis Cd's, supplements, and all manner of nicotine delivery substitutes. Ones which aside from the new electric cigarettes on the market, I once tried every one of.

You see, just like big Americans desperate to loose weight, every smoker knows that they are sticking a middle finger up at their long term health.

It wasn't however, until a night in 2008 that someone actually told me how to really kick the habit for good.

You see, I'd been quit for just over six months and although that might sound great, it wasn't. Something would always happen around the sixth month mark. Either I'd crash the car, or me and my boyfriend would have an argument; or as it was this time, I'd wind up fired.

Actually, I'd been laid off in the morning, and me and my boyfriend had broke up in the afternoon, so you could call that one a bit of a double whammy.

Anyway, by the evening I'd decided to visit my local seven eleven, get a hot dog and some chicken wings, fill the car up ready for the next day, buy a couple of packets of cigarettes, and then hit the bar across the road from my apartment.

To a lot of people that might sound trashy. But to be honest I'm just being real here and it's not like I was looking to get picked up. Rather, I was just really angry. You see, sometimes life does stuff to you and you know what? Sometimes there isn't even time to get upset.

In fact, by mid afternoon that day, I'd just felt like walking in to the middle of the highway near where I live, and screaming, "are you kidding me?"

Anyway, I ended up in this bar and even though Halloween had already passed, they still had pumpkin flavored beer on tap, so I grabbed a stool feeling like I was the only person who didn't know who everyone else was, and settled in for an hour with forty little white and yellow sticks to support my spirits.

Not long after however, I struck up conversation with some old guy called James, and you know what? He was exactly what I needed.

Of course, I'm not going to bore you with the full length of our conversation. James did however, tell me two things that I'll remember forever, the first of which I've already told you. - This being that anyone anywhere is only ever five minutes away from the rest of their life yada yada, and that what's running through anyone's mind in that five minutes isn't anyone's business but their own.

The second however, was to me at least the most profound. You see, as I told James about my notorious six month quitting crash and burns, and how the present one was really taking the pee, he said, "honey, let me just stop you right there."

"You see, you're going to have to get your head around something at some point," he said looking at me knowingly. "And that something is that once you're a smoker, you're always a smoker."

"You can go," he said, "the rest of your whole life without one, but the simple truth is that you're always going to want one."

46

Then James, the friend who I've never seen since, suggested that I simply smoke my fill for the evening, before leaving whatever I didn't finish on the bar when I left. "Because you can always get back on track tomorrow."

Moreover, that's exactly what I did. And because I'd already gone six months without them and knew that I could do it, it really wasn't that difficult.

You see, what I'd always done previously, was aim for something which wasn't actually achievable. This being a state of physical being in which I wouldn't ever want or need to smoke ever again.

What I therefore decided to try and achieve instead, was something that I knew I could achieve very easily, so long as I didn't smoke for more than a day at a time every couple of months or so. - This something being a smoker who's simply making a decision not to smoke.

In fact, when I told this to my mum who's been battling to quit cigarettes on and off for twenty years at least, she almost broke down in tears.

You see, it's true. Once you're a smoker you really always are a smoker. I've since went eighteen months without a cigarette, and although on most days I could get to the point where it didn't even cross my mind, I did underneath it all, want nothing more in some moments, than to suck on a freshly lit

Marlboro, breathe it in real real deep and exhale it slowly, with perhaps even an audible, "ahhhh."

Further, it works differently for everyone. Some people can go a week, some people can go a month, and some people can go whole months at a time. But when you take away the sense of failure and can practice enough self restraint to put at least seven or thirty days between your next packet of cigarettes, it makes a hell of a difference.

You feel better about yourself physically. You feel better about yourself emotionally via your replacing your "I'm such a failure," inferiority complex, with one that says that actually you're in control. And by and large it's a hell of a lot easier for someone to put down the cigarettes finally, when they know that the decision isn't dependent on them doing so forever.

Of course, non-smokers and smokers who have been quit for years will cry foul at this assertion.

Indeed, my fiend Robyn knows fine well that I've had less than ten cartons of cigarettes since 2008, but she still categorizes my occasional return to the habit every six months, as a complete failure. In fact, she often treats it like some irrecoverable moral tragedy, and I find that rather amusing.

You see, I don't harass her when her latest diet regimen implodes spectacularly, and she practically mauls her way through buckets of chicken and cartons of fries and gravy.

Nor in fact, do I ever say, "Jesus Robyn, how fat are you actually trying to get?"

However, here's my point. If you like to binge and eat all the wrong kinds of food, you're always going to be like that.

You can drop three hundred pounds, have surgery to take all the excess skin away and make you beautiful, and you can even make a career for yourself as a celebrity. You want your perfect world, you got it.

You are however, always going to want to race to TGI Fridays every once in a while and gorge your way through Fridays Pick Three For All.

Likewise, you are going to run into Subway occasionally and order a six inch steak egg and cheese.

Rather however, than feel bad about that when you do, and rather than think that you have failed yourself or anyone else in the process; just realize such occurrences for what they are. These being mere moments when you've let the real you out. The opening and closing of a pressure valve, without which you might have exploded completely.

Then, simply make sure to reassert control over yourself again tomorrow.

You see, here's the kicker. Your mouth isn't just something that you eat or smoke with. It's a sensory organ in it's own right and in many respects it's the most powerful one.

Babies for instance, gargle, and spit, and chew, and always have to have something in their mouths, not because they are always hungry or need a pacifier.

Rather, it's been proven that babies and young children actually explore the world around them with their mouths. They familiarize themselves with it's textures, pliability and tastes orally, and with this being the case, our senses of taste and smell, are often hard wired into our emotional memories.

Hence why sometimes you can smell something that takes you right back for a moment to your grandparents or your parents house in your childhood. And hence why when we loose somebody, we keep their clothes and toiletry sets, just so as to create a sense that they are somehow still close.

This being the case, and although you probably don't know it, your overeating (especially if you have been big since childhood or adolescence) is hard wired into the very emotional centers of your being.

In fact, for all intensive purposes many overweight Americans have actually permanently associated their respective senses of emotional happiness with food.

Moreover, although this might sound far fetched it really isn't. People start to get depressed when they start putting on weight. Then they comfort eat to counter this depression. Then they get bigger because of the extra eating, and so the cycle continues.

The synaptic pathways that we subsequently build between our sense of happiness and our sense's of taste, do not however, simply uncouple just because we decide to start juicing or practicing intermittent fasting.

Rather, just like the pathways that take you right back to your childhood when you smell certain aromas, they are always going to be part of you, and you are always going to associate food with an emotional sense of pleasure and happiness.

You therefore need to accept that being big, (even if you get real small) is always going to be a part of you. You need to accept that you will fall off the wagon from time to time. And you need to accept that people around you will quite possibly feel like they have a right to give you a hard time about that.

If however, you can brush the crumbs off your midriff once you're done chewing your way through a 10oz steak and lobster tail at your favorite diner, and know that at most such an experience can only ever be a monthly or six monthly one, you're not being a weak person, you're being someone who is in control of their own life.

Further, when we diet in the conventional sense and we either abandon certain foods that we like or severely restrict how much we have of them, all we do is give rise to emotional conflict cycles within ourselves.

Let's say that you have decided to abstain indefinitely from chocolate. You see, the problem here is that for what is likely a significant length of time by now, you've actually come to psychologically associate eating chocolate with emotional pleasure.

This being the case, taking it away and telling yourself that you can't ever have it again, subsequently makes you feel depressed and angry with yourself. And you know what? It's precisely when you feel like that, that you're likely to throw in the towel with whatever diet regimen that you're trying to stick to.

Telling yourself instead however, that you can only have chocolate once a week, or once a month, providing that you stick to the diet and exercise regimen that you have promised yourself that you will, reaffirms psychologically chocolates standing in your life as something emotionally satisfying. In this case a reward.

Of course, don't get me wrong, cutting down is going to suck, and I was deadly serious when I told you to empty your kitchen of anything and everything artificial.

However, before we start any kind of diet we need to come to terms with why we are the way that we are. Further, although I stand by my assertion already that our food being jam packed full of artificial toxins and GMO ingredients is a significant, if not the most significant contributor to obesity and being over weight in America; we also need to take psychological responsibility for what we have done to ourselves.

Indeed, diet books that blame America's weight on wheat, red meat and dairy, do nothing other than help America project the blame for its weight onto outside and by and large unaccountable third parties.

What we need to do instead however, is understand that we are not just responsible for what we have put into our bodies in order for us to get this way, but that we have an underlying psychological and emotional relationship with our food. A relationship that we need to recondition before we can really ever set about making permanent and positive changes to our respective lives and diets.

STARTING OVER

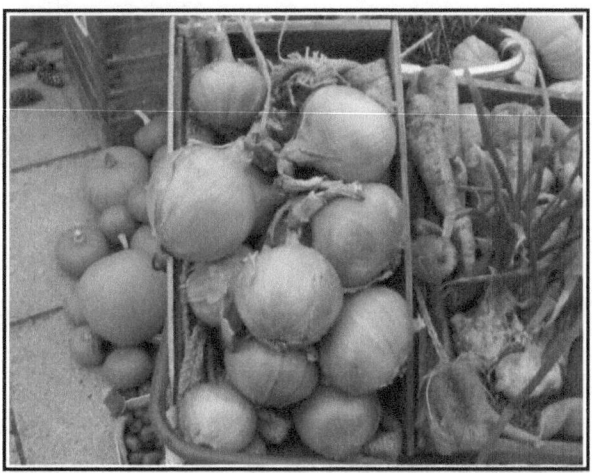

So, you've ditched pretty much everything that you had in your refrigerator and you're thinking, well what now?[7]

In fact, when you strip down food to its basics, i.e. a selection of loose fruit and vegetables, a hunk of raw meat, and maybe a packet of dried peas or lentils, it pretty much looks like nothing.

Now however, you're going to have to sit down and make a list. One detailing as many of your favorite foods as you can think of. Do not however, populate

7   IMAGE COURTESY OF PAUL38 AT WWW.SXC.HU

this list with things like Cheeto's, Betty Crocker Mash Potatoes, or Butterball Turkey Burgers. You are done buying brands.

I want you to list actual meals that you like. Meals like lasagna, and stir fried chicken.

I want you to list different things that you like having for breakfast, different things that you like having for lunch, and I even want you to list what kind of things you like having for desert.

Further, I don't want you to stop until you have at least twenty main evening meal ideas written down in front of you.

Now however, comes the difficult part.

You see, with the regimen that I want to advocate here, you're allowed everything on the list you just wrote. The only problem is that you're not allowed to order out, you're not allowed to buy whatever it is ready made, and you're certainly not allowed to use any ready in five minute packet ingredients like hamburger helper.

Let's take a burger and fries for example. You see, when it's ready you can smother that burger in as much mayonnaise as you want and you can spice them fries up with as much ketchup as you like.

The thing is, you're going to have to cut those fries

in the first place from actual potatoes. Then you're going to have to oven bake them for yourself with lashings of extra virgin olive oil.

Indeed, you're going to have to season (with real herbs) your mince meat before forming it into beef patties. And as well as baking your own bread buns, you're even going to have to make up your own ketchup and mayonnaise.

In fact, let's get a little more adventurous here and let's say that you have lasagna and garlic bread on your list.

You see, once again you're going to have to bake your own bread. Then you're going to have to make up three batches of sauce, and then you're going to have to layer and bake your own lasagna. And yeah that might sound easier, but you're probably forgetting that your favorite brand of pasata or pre-chopped tomatoes, as well as any cream (unless you can get your hands on an organic carton) is now strictly off limits.

This being the case, you're going to have to make maybe the first authentic lasagna that you have ever eaten. You're going to have to chop and simmer your tomatoes into a thick red sauce. You're going to have to beat your own egg yolks and organic cream into white sauce, and you're going to have to make your own cheese sauce and topping.

Moreover, let me just make this clear from the start. You are going to mess up. It's going to take some people a full week, maybe even a full month before they can get their bread to rise, never mind bake anything that looks even remotely like a baguette or a bread bun.

Commitment and steadfastness in the face of such trial and error is however, fundamental in setting both your mind and body on course to a healthier and happier future.

Bread lovers will find for example, that they really need to set aside a whole day each week in order to really bake as much as they need for the next seven days.

Further, home baked bread won't last more than a day or so even in the refrigerator, (until you have mastered the process) before it starts to go stale.

This being the case, you're probably best freezing as much as you can, as well as leaving a couple of bars of dough in the refrigerator that you can bake any time.

What's more, if you have a particularly busy schedule, you're going to want to bake as much as possible of everything you might want to eat over the next week, that has a substantial preparation time.

For peace of mind for example, you might want to make sure to always have a couple of meat loafs or something ready. No one's life after all, ever runs as steadily as they would like it to week to week.

Of course, you can also take things much slower.

In fact, what I used to do in the beginning, is cook up a huge pot of chicken soup literally swimming in root vegetables and mushrooms, and have this simmering away whilst I tried to get my head around different bread and flat bread recipes.

Being single at the time I always made about a gallon. Then, with there being enough for the next day and sometimes even the day after that, I had more than enough time to try out different desert and snack recipes.

Moreover, making different soups from scratch is a great way to actually start refortifying your body with the nutrients that it needs, whilst also having something perfectly suited to eating with your first home made bread selections.

In fact, for at least the first couple of months I was pretty much rotating between chicken and vegetable broth, broccoli and Stilton soup, (my personal favorite by the way) and a really thick Hungarian beef goulash.

After this however, not only was I comfortable

making my own bread, cereal bars and all the basic pasta sauces that I liked. But rather, I was starting to really enjoy learning how to cook and prepare more complex recipe ideas.

Of course, I burnt sauces and I ruined my first batches of oat, honey and millet bars. However, as my initial inhibitions and my sense of 'I really don't know where to start,' was steadily replaced by a certain level of working experience, I started to really feel at home in my own kitchen.

I started to experiment by putting a cup full of vegetable stock, along with onions, chunks of carrot and everything, into a batch of dough instead of just plain old warm water.

Further, I remembered how someone had told me once that a lot of gateaux' that you see, in specialist cake shops, actually have a ton of mayonnaise in them to keep them moist. As such, I whisked together a couple of egg yolks and olive oil one day and hey presto, I'd just found a way to extend the shelf life of my own baked goods!

One thing that I did learn quite quickly however, was that it's pretty pointless buying a stack of recipe books to get you started. Don't get me wrong, I still have a whole shelf full, and so I'm not saying that that they are completely useless.

However, I never and I mean never, seemed to have

many of the things that I needed to finish a single meal.

I wouldn't have lemon grass or I wouldn't have cumin. Then, I'd go through this kind of mental process in which I felt like a real looser, because clearly everyone else in America must obviously know what all these things are and always have a spice rack full of them.

In the end therefore, I decided that if I was ever going to be cooking something special for someone, I'd consult the recipe first, and nip to the store to make sure that I had everything that I needed.

For day to day cooking however, I'd simply print out a few recipes that I had found on the Internet. One's which either I already had everything that I needed to prepare, or in the worst case would just have to improvise slightly.

Fast forwarding then, to three months into my new regimen, not only could I say that I was clean of GMO's, refined sugar, unnatural chemicals, and even metal particulates such as aluminum. But more than that, I felt great and was proud enough to boast to anyone willing to hear it, just what exactly I could do by then in the kitchen.

Indeed, I realized when I finally mastered baking bread properly, that I'd actually never tasted anything like it before. I mean yeah it was bread, but it was thicker, tasted more like bread and was about five times as substantial.

This being the case, I toyed for a while with taking some to work and handing it around. However, in respect of the fact that it tastes best when fresh out of the oven, I thought hey, why don't I just invite some people around for dinner?

In fact, this is when I knew that I was on to something with ditching so called 'convenient' food. You see, I wasn't any thinner. Maybe I'd lost a pound or two, but to be honest I put weighing myself everyday behind me, when I was still picking up and putting down cigarette cartons.

I did however, feel fantastic. I was loving cooking. I was loving this new energy I had coursing through my body, and although I didn't put two and two together immediately, this new energy was coming from two distinct places.

First, my metabolism was waking up. My body was saying, "hey, we've actually got bread here! Not rubber elasticity compounds, not 2-methylimidazole or 4-methylimidazole, not even potassium bromate, just bread!"

"Look!" My GMO punctured lower gut cells were then shouting, "we've got real food coming through here too! No corn that metabolizes as the soil bacteria Bacillus Thuringiensis, and decimates our enzyme and friendly bacteria count. We've even got real, non mechanically rendered meat!"

The second thing that was happening, was that where previously I, just like many Americans had associated food with pleasure, I was now associating food not just with pleasure, but with pride and a want of sharing my individual experience in eating it.

Of course, we all like going out for dinner, and even though it's sometimes awkward, most of us do still like gathering together to eat with our families once in a while. But this was different. I felt like I wanted to invite people into my home and serve them my cooking, knowing that I would be able to tell them exactly what was in every bite.

I wanted people to experience bread for the first time just like me. And it's not that I wanted to show off. Rather, I simply wanted to share what I had found.

"Here," I wanted to shout. "Here's America like it used to be, how it used to taste and smell. Now come, gather round, and see what you've been missing for half a century!"

Moreover, when you re-find the heart and soul of good wholesome honest cooking and food preparation, you re-find the heart and soul of why it's so ingrained in us psychologically and emotionally to start with.

We may for example, have had the pseudo political myth of the first Thanksgiving handed down to us. However, what we often forget is that the Mayflower pilgrims would have actually perished completely in 1620, if it wasn't for the Wampanoag Indians showing them how to plant, gather and preserve food in America in the first place.

Likewise, what was the most important thing that Jesus wanted to do, even though he new that he'd likely be executed the next day? - He simply wanted to break bread with those closest to him.

Food if you like, unites us. Moreover, I'm not talking about the way it unites us at The Cheesecake Factory or PF Chang's. In fact, perhaps you can't really understand what I'm talking about until you have experienced it for yourself. But there is something really special about bringing something to a table for your friends and your loved ones to enjoy.

You see, food isn't just fuel for our bodies. Yeah, it keeps us going however, on a molecular and even a genetic level, the food we eat is absorbed into becoming new and replacement parts of our very being.

Our grandparents in fact, hit the nail on the head

when they tried to tell us that we are what we eat.

You see, living inside every single cell in our body, there are these little things called organelles which act like tiny cranes at tiny ports, lifting what they need from the food that's continually being absorbed into our bloodstream.

With what they lift out, they then set about manufacturing new cells, whilst simultaneously organizing vitamins, minerals and essential fats, into whatever the existing cell might require to fend off disease and free-radicals, and in general just stay healthy.

This being the case, when I serve a guest at my table whatever food I've prepared, I'm not just filling them up with the nutrient equivalent of gasoline. Rather, I'm serving that person nutrient rich, completely additive free food, prepared with real affection; in full knowledge that even though I might never see that person again, that food will be part of them forever.

The idea then, of ever again serving my present boyfriend with a microwave dinner that's riddled with genetically modified corn starch and preservatives, nothing short of disgusts me.

What disgusts me even more however, is the fact that I spent thirty years of my life eating that very same kind of preprepared crap, without ever giving it a second thought.

Moreover, just think about what I'm trying to give you here. Yes I'm giving you one hell of a challenge, hell, I'm even telling you than not only will it not be easy, but that you will fall off the wagon at some point.

However, I'm also giving you a ticket to better health and better emotional balance in your life.

Is therefore, my saying that you just have to cook everything that you want to eat from scratch, such a big price to pay?

Of course, there are going to be people here who say, "hey aren't you going to give us a recipe for bread at least?" And to that I'm just going to say sorry, but you really have to do this for yourself.

In fact, if I was writing this just because I want to make a fast buck, I would have just spent a week on the Internet rewriting a hundred exotic smoothy recipes.

Moreover, you're not me. If I just supplied you here with recipes for everything that I eat every week, this simply wouldn't work. You would get bored. Gastronomically you would feel limited and start pining for your favorite barbecue chicken wings.

This being the case, you would likely stick with the

basic principles of the regimen that I want to advocate for a week or two. But after that you would likely do the same thing that you did after doing the south beach diet, or that two week juicing run that you did last summer, and simply start looking for a more practical way to loose weight.

So sorry, if you like having eggs Benedict for breakfast, you're simply going to have to find the recipe for yourself, find a way to make it appropriate to the given regimen, and then take it for a whirl on your own.

Just stick to the five rules below:

- Do not consume any artificial ingredients at all. This means bread, dairy products and anything genetically modified. Because most States don't have GMO labeling legislature, you will have to find a way to determine what produce in you local supermarket is genetically modified and what isn't, but it is possible.
- Milk, flour, eggs, pasta and anything else you use for baking must be organic. It's more expensive, but buying organic milk puts a stop to you ingesting bovine growth hormones. Similarly, flour and pasta bought organically protects you from GMO contamination, whilst organic eggs protect you from poultry antibiotics and vaccines (which are inclusive of viruses and liquid

mercury).
- Don't use refined sugar in any of your cooking. (Try buying organic sugar or using molasses). And if there's anything on a label that you can't pronounce DON'T BUY IT. (Try buying organic sugar or using molasses).
- Prepare all your own food without any exception. If this seems too difficult just think about it this way: Out of a thousand generations before you, you'll be the first that couldn't figure out how to feed yourself.
- Research, Research, Research!

Meanwhile, keep in mind throughout the development of your new life and food experience, that you're not doing anyone's diet or anyone else's copyrighted regimen. This is simply the bare bones of a lifestyle choice, that the best part about undertaking is that you can sculpt it to fit with and be as unique as your very own personality.

ASPARTAME

"Oh come on it's just a soda." And, "you know I think that you're taking this way to far, it's only Wendy's for Chrissakes!" And: "You know I saw this thing on the news that said that GMO is actually nutritionally better than non-GMO produce."[8]

These and a thousand other such statements are going to come at you from all sides once you do decide to take personal control back over your own diet and well being.

---

8   IMAGE COURTESY OF MATTHIJS VAN HEERIKHUIZE AT WWW.VANHEERIKHUIZE.NL

In fact, even though I've lost a hundred pounds since I changed my own diet and lifestyle, and even though I've since then had no problem maintaining a weight and body shape that I'm comfortable with, people like my friend Robyn simply wont merit this accomplishment as being attributable to my choice of diet and lifestyle.

It's insane. If I'd achieved the same results by following a Jenny Craig regimen, I'd be equivocal to my friends personal hero. However, because the method by which I have lost weight isn't emotionally or practically convenient for people like my friend Robyn, she and others routinely try to ridicule me for it.

Moreover, it is even the case that some people directly attack this lifestyle choice. Hell, I even found myself wondering at one point, (and still do for that matter) if this is what it must be like to be gay in modern America.

You see, we all seem to run around patting each other on the back for having free will and the like. However, the minute that many Americans are presented with someone who for whatever reason, has decided to live their life differently to theirs; they seem to feel the need to attack that person.

Let's take a real day at work which I had recently.

You see, I work in the administration department of

a plumbing company, and even though it's just a desk job, I really do like my work.

Whereas once however, me and my co-workers used to eat out for lunch everyday, I had to break from that dynamic when I started eating food that I could be 100% certain of what was actually in it.

Of course, this wasn't a problem, not at first anyway. I'd been bothered by periodic bouts of IBS for months and everyone just assumed that I was doing some kind of medically advised diet.

When however, it became obvious that my diet and lifestyle change was permanent, a couple of people that I work with started to suggest that I might actually have an eating disorder, or be in some way emotionally unbalanced.

Production of a packed lunch usually remedied this assertion however, a little while later people started to actually verbally bully me. "Hey Chelsea do you wanna grab a Chinese with us? Oh sorry, I forgot you're too good for stuff like that..." And yeah that sounds real childish, but when it happens almost everyday it does start to effect you.

Anyway, I'd always let this go until about a month ago when this new girl started in our department. I was showing her the ropes and we were hitting it off real well. When lunch time came around however, this girl turned to ask if I was coming with everyone to a sandwich bar near by, only for one of my co-workers to turn around and say, "you know what don't even go there, Chelsea's so paranoid about what she eats that she won't even drink soda."

And that pushed it too far for me.

You see, I was actually going to be working as this girls supervisor, and not only was this statement said in such a way that it undermined me in a psychological sense, but it introduced into my workplaces dynamic, the idea that from now on anybody new coming to work in the department will be orientated as usual, before being told, "oh and hey, this is Chelsea and she's different."

Rather however, than lodge an official complaint, I've simply decided to look for a new job.

Moreover, don't get me wrong, there are more people that I work with that are fantastic. People who I have round to dinner occasionally, and people who I go out for drinks with just like everyone else.

In fact, on a number of occasions, a guy who I work with has had me dissect in excruciating detail, my bread making process, as he stares in awe at the home made sun dried tomato bread rolls which I often take to work with me.

Likewise, I actually met my current boyfriend via

me turning his initial attempt to invite me out for dinner, into me inviting him over to my place for something to eat.

And not only have my mother and my brother actually embraced my dietary regimen for themselves, (albeit not as strictly) but I've visibly watched them be transformed from tired, pasty looking people, into people glowing with renewed health and vitality.

Further, although she routinely attacks my cooking and diet regimen, me and my friend Robyn will still be friends for the rest of our lives.

I am not however, breaking down my main personal relationships here, in an effort to prepare you for your own being ridiculed or dismissed by people in your immediate work and social circles.

Rather, I'm demonstrating the fact that many American's simply can't accept the fact, that most of what they eat and drink every day might actually be bad for them. You can talk until you're blue in the face but they simply won't get it, and quite frankly they don't want to get it.

You see, Americans often seem to try and avoid taking on board easily verifiable facts, just because those facts are emotionally inconvenient.

People in general tend to agree for example, that

lawyers, big industry corporatists, and state department officials are quite easily corruptible. Hell, I even read somewhere recently that 80% of Americans believe that 9/11 was an inside job.

However, when it comes to the food that we eat every day, people simply don't want to believe that they are for all intensive purposes being systematically poisoned for profit by such very individuals.

Take aspartame for example. Aspartame and aspartame derived artificial sweeteners are everywhere in the average American diet.

Almost all soda and fruit squash, and every brand of diet soda that you will find sold anywhere is packed full of the stuff.

This being the case, Americans by and large believe that aspartame, just like everything else that they eat and drink, has been rigorously tested by both the FDA, and the people who produce it in the first place.

Sadly however, this simply isn't the case. In fact, almost immediately after first being approved for human consumption in 1974, this approval was rescinded due to diketopiperazine in aspartame being found to cause brain tumors.

Not however, to be thwarted so easily, G.D. Searle,

aspartames original inventor, then simply waited seven years until things like deliberately falsified test results were forgotten about, before having aspartame approved by a new FDA director.

Tellingly, Dr Arthur H. Hayes, the director in question, then resigned three months later, in order to take up a $1000 a day role with Burson Marsteller, the public relations firm for Nutrasweet.

The fact remains therefore, that not only has aspartame never been fully vetted for its safety, but laboratory tests since then have shown that aspartame doesn't just cause brain tumors. Rather, the substance has been shown to cause brain tumors., breast tumors., uterine tumors., and pancreatic tumors.

Further, animals fed individual components of aspartame, have in turn had young which have developed into morbidly obese and sexually dysfunctional adults. Whilst in humans, aspartame has been shown to exasperate and induce onset of:

Epilepsy, Parkinson's Disease, Alzheimer's, Multiple Sclerosis, Chronic Fatigue, Syndrome, Lymphoma, Fibromyalgia, Mental Retardation, Birth Defects, Diabetes, Hypoglycemia, Graves Disease, Heart Disease, Lung Disease, Liver Disease, Kidney Disease, Arthritis, Blindness, Tinnitus, Carpal Tunnel Syndrome, and Muniere's Disease.

As well, that is, as a host of other rare and so hard to diagnose disorders, that aspartame has been called a systemic toxin. One which over time adversely effects every organ and biological process in the human body.

Moreover, millions of Americans have already been adversely effected by aspartame. Suspiciously however, all lawsuits which have ever been brought against Nutrasweet and/or the FDA, have simply been dropped or settled out of court.

In fact, the Supreme Court itself has since simply refused to hear a case brought against the FDA by the consumer rights crusader James Turner, in which Turner was petitioning for aspartame to be made illegal due to the substance violating The Delaney Clause. (One which states that no substance can be approved for human consumption by the FDA, which is shown to cause cancer).

What is more, in 1995, the United States began introducing laws to directly curb such suits from ever getting so far in the first place, by making it illegal under the Agricultural Defamation Act, for anyone to ever say anything disparaging about a perishable food product.

This then, is the long and short of what you need to get your head around. The FDA isn't a body which looks out for your best interests. The FDA is there so that big companies can lobby to be legally permitted to poison you.

You see, it's not like someone discovers a new kind of potato and goes to the FDA to get it approved for sale and human consumption. Rather, the science division of a generic frozen pizza manufacturer might find that the food manufacture in question, could make its pizza's look and taste cheesier whilst actually using less cheese, if only they could use artificial wonder compound 537.

The scientists and lawyers for this frozen pizza manufacturer subsequently go to the FDA and say "hey, could you just authorize artificial wonder compound 537 for human consumption? - You know, its that industrial lubricant people usually use in heavy goods vehicles, but we did some tests and it's perfectly safe for humans to eat. It does tend to give cancer to any other animal that eats it, but we don't think that's anything to worry about."

A few words, lobbying dollars and job offers later, and artificial wonder compound 537 is boxed and ready to go in frozen pizzas in Walmart's everywhere. One's which because they are made with 50% less cheese, are advertised perversely as **50% FAT FREE!**

Moreover, I'm sorry if you find this pessimistic or ideologically opposed to what you presently believe, in regard to the food you eat and feed your children. But this is not my point of view. These are simply facts which you haven't taken the time to familiarize yourself with before, and it's not just aspartame.

Indeed, the monosodium glutamate or MSG, that you will find in everything from your bottles of ketchup, to your kids confectionery, and those turkey burgers you like so much, is actually a proven neuro-toxin. One which just like aspartame, has been proven to cause brain tumors., and as such has been banned from use in baby food since the 60's.

What is more, MSG only got onto the American dinner table as a flavor enhancer, after the US military realized in 1948, that the compound was being added to Japanese soldiers ration packs.

Similarly, it's been known since the 1970's that sodium nitrate used to help preserve bacon, hot dogs and almost all processed fish and meat products, is inherently carcinogenic.

However, it was lobbying by big industry food manufacturers at the same time, which saw efforts to ban the substance fail miserably.

Isn't there an alternative to using sodium nitrate you might ask? Why of course! The only problem is that sodium nitrate has this nifty side effect of making old, poor quality cuts of meat, appear red and fresh and appetizing. And because no other preservative acts so favorably cosmetically, many big food manufacturers simply can't bare the idea of giving it up just yet.

So here it is, I'm just someone who thought gosh, here are three products that I'm consuming every day and you know what? I'm not happy with either my body or my overall health, why don't I just try and remove these from my diet for a while and see what happens?

Moreover, how dietary advice given by doctors and renowned health and fitness experts around the world, routinely omits to mention the proven and physiologically damning effects of such everyday additives, strikes me as nothing more than criminal.

America is big fat and unhealthy. It's got big fat and unhealthy whilst consuming vast amounts of substances laced with things proven to make people big fat and unhealthy, and me pointing out the fact makes me socially reprehensible?

Come on.

Do your own freaking research America. Get your head out your "oh but I just don't have the time and my kids just love cheese strings," big fat behind and wake up to what you're actually putting in your kids lunch boxes!

I mean if the young of rodents fed the same

aspartic acid from your favorite soft drink, are scientifically proven to be more prone to obesity, docility, and sexual dysfunction, couldn't there be a link there between, oh I don't know, America's fatter than ever before, and more autistic than ever before children?

And hey, whilst we're harping on about gun control and prescribing Ritalin to millions of supposedly attention deficit stricken American teenagers, why is no one asking why a substance originally put in Japanese soldiers rations to make them more hyper and aggressive, is now a staple in almost every Americans day to day diet?

Moreover, when I hear that one in three women are likely to develop cancer, rather than prostrate myself before E! Entertainment as it pays tribute to Angelina Jolie having a preventative double mastectomy, I sit thinking gosh, wouldn't it be great if someone like her could start a movement to have sodium nitrate taken out of the food chain?

You see, the science is there. Neither me or advocates of organic produce, or people trying to bring America's GMO industry to account, are people with personal vendettas against the food industry in general. Hell, when you educate yourself it gets relatively easy to side step all their toxic products in the first place.

Rather, I just think to myself, "you know what

Chelsea? You used to eat all that junk too, and no one ever tried to tell you what it actually was that you were doing to your body, so maybe it would be nice to try and help someone else."

You see, as much as I would love to, I simply can't furnish you with a way to loose a pound a day or drop six dress sizes in six weeks. What I can do though, is say hey America, you wanna get slim, stay trim, and feel great in the long term? Well this is what worked for me, and here's why.

Furthermore, even if you are still ideologically undecided, in 15,000 words so far I've demonstrated how there are known carcinogens in the bread you buy, coal tar derived toxic colorings in everything from your bread to your favorite brand of macaroni, fire retardants in your fish, neuro-toxins and obesity causing artificial flavor enhancers in your soda, and cancer causing nitrates in any processed meats that you might like. Now does that really sound okay to you?

Moreover, I'm sorry. But as far as I'm concerned yeah, I could save time by spending a bit longer in Safeway and stocking up on bread, pasta and pizza that's already been made for me.

Do however, I think that that foods convenient?

Hell no!

~ It's Not The Freaking Wheat America ~

THE GMO DEBACLE

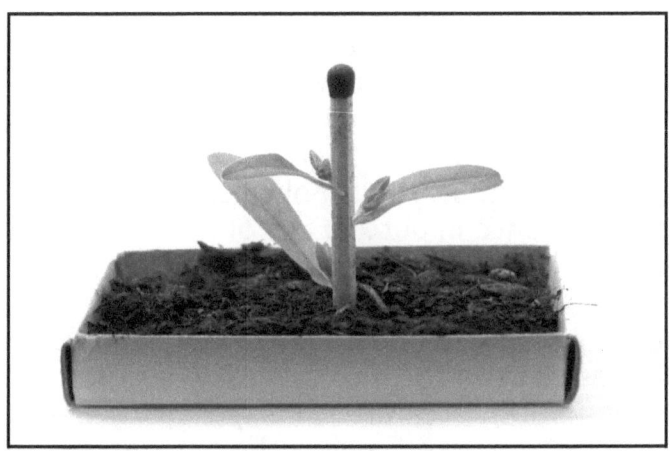

I used to love corn. I'd always have a bag of frozen corn on the cob in the freezer, ready to take out and have with a grilled chicken sandwich or something.[9]

Moreover, one of the most heavenly scents in the world to me, was the scent of corn syrup circulating in the air at PF Chang's.

I haven't however, touched corn in any way shape or form, for nearly eighteen months at present. In fact, I won't even buy organic. You see, although I was aware of the fact that most of America's corn is

---

9   IMAGE COURTESY OF HUMUSAK2 AT WWW.SXC.HU

genetically modified, I wasn't aware until a year and a half ago, that GMO contamination can now be measured in almost all organic corn fields in America.

Of course, that's not to say that all of America's organic corn is actually genetically modified. However, cross contamination does occur, and because I'm aware of what GMO technology actually does to us, I've simply made a decision, not to take a chance in putting any of it in my body. Not even by accident.

You see, genetic modification of our food does not take place in the form of scientists surrounded by supercomputers, carefully inserting genes into predetermined fixed points in a plant, or as is becoming the case also, animals DNA.

Rather, genes that a corporation would like to insert into a specific plant or animal, are mixed with cocktails of enzymes and viruses, before being bonded to nano sized particles of gold, and then literally shot with what is called a 'gene gun,' at a culture of cells belonging to the organism being modified.

The nano gold particles subsequently punch holes in the original organisms DNA, and the viruses and enzymes quickly get to work patching those holes with the new genes that American agribusinesses want to see introduced, so as to give the plant or animal in question, some new commercially desirable genetic traits.

In short therefore, for any DNA that is inserted into the target organism, some indigenous DNA is irreparably destroyed. Further, because of the method of delivery of the genes being transferred, no scientist or supercomputer knows what DNA will be destroyed, or where the new genes will actually be inserted.

Genetic modification, is if you like, merely a game of Russian roulette. Moreover, with this being the case, fundamental questions are raised.

You see, plants and animals do acquire new genetic traits from generation to generation. Humans have capitalized on this knowledge for hundreds of years via selectively breeding livestock and selectively pollinating agricultural crops.

Never however, do genes naturally cross species barriers. In fact, even the most un-complex of amoebas are designed in such a way as to prevent the absorption or accidental transfer of anything other than amoeba stamped and certified DNA.

This being the case, genetically modified crops are completely new to the worlds five or so billion year old ecosystem, and any scientist not financially affiliated with the GMO industry will gladly inform you that no one anywhere, no matter their political, academic or social standing, can honestly tell you what these crops will do, either when introduced to the environment or for that matter into the human body.

As it stands however, the FDA in the United States has stipulated that GMO crops are inherently safe.

This safety is proven, the FDA asserts, by animal GMO feeding studies, which the GMO industry itself has funded, overseen, and personally collated the data of.

What the FDA refuses to acknowledge however, is the fact that genetic modification firms themselves flatly refuse to carry out any study for longer than thirty days. Moreover, because GMO plants and seeds are classed as containing propriety information, GMO producers often refuse to allow independent scientists to carry out their own independent research.

Tellingly however, not only has it been revealed in recent years, that employees of Monsanto, one of America's biggest GMO producers, themselves demand only to be served organic produce in Monsanto's own workplace cafeterias. But also, the few scientists whom have done independent GMO feeding studies, have all found that over the course of a full lifetime, rodents fed GMO produce become obese, docile, and susceptible to developing cancers of almost every variety.

Of course, such scientists are often paraded as charlatans before the world however, it is worth keeping in mind, that such denunciations ultimately come in the first place from a food industry and an FDA, whom have together since the 1950's, decided that it is perfectly safe to put titanium oxide in baked goods to make them appear whiter, and similarly A-okay, to call beaver anal gland juice a 'natural flavoring' when it's used as raspberry or vanilla flavoring in your favorite ice cream.

The Hungarian (though at the time UK based) scientist Árpád Pusztai, was for example, fired in 1998, and banned by the British government from speaking about his work, due simply to him stating publicly, that in the course of his study on genetically modified potatoes, he had witnessed damage to both the intestine and autoimmune systems of rats being fed such.

Further, although Pusztai has been vilified by American and British press and agribusiness interests, his work and others, is often cited by independent scientists, 828 of whom from around the world, have since 2000, been petitioning all world governments to in the least case temporarily suspend GMO production and cultivation for a period of five years.

This being the absolute minimum amount of time necessary in order to carry out legitimate and independently verifiable research into the inherent safety or not, of human GMO consumption. As well as on the effect of genetically modified organisms being unleashed into the earth's environment.

Now if I was the FDA, and on one side I had a corporation insisting that its 30 day rodent consumption trials of GMO are enough to guarantee such organisms safety, and on the other I had 828 independent scientists from around the world saying, "hold on, can we just have five years to really look at this a little bit more closely?" I know who I'd give the benefit of the doubt.

However, not granting such a five year hiatus shouldn't really surprise. You see, there is enough verified research already, which suggests that GMO's are the last thing that people should be eating.

Independent researchers in Canada for instance, have already proved that in the process of digesting GM soy, the insecticide producing genes inserted into the soy in the lab actually migrate into the DNA of bacteria permanently resident in the human gut.

This being the case, bacteria in peoples own bodies start continuously producing insecticides which then start systematically effecting our bodies, to the extent that a child born to a woman who has eaten GM soy, will also be born not only with this toxin already inside them, but with the bacteria that makes it inside them also.

And let's just clarify here, this isn't anyone's theory or idle speculation, this is a verifiable scientific fact.

As for that matter, is the fact that in the years since GMO crops have been branded fit for human consumption, chronic disease in America has jumped from affecting 7% of the overall population to 13%. Food allergies have in the same time sky-rocketed, and even the American Academy of Emergency Medicine has attempted to advise people to pre-emptively avoid GMO produce, rather than wait around for someone to come and say definitively whether it's safe or not.

Moreover, with farmers around the world now starting to report lower fertility, gastric complaints and even gross birth defects in animal herds being fed GMO corn and soy, it really is only a matter of time before the lid flies off the GMO debate.

Like in the case of thalidomide in the late 1950's however, no one is likely to start taking on board the full implications of the FDA's oversight and blatant disregard of independent science, until American children start being born with the same deformities presently being seen in pigs and cattle in Europe.

Of course, this is a very contentious subject. People however, need to divorce themselves from the idea that their American identity is somehow intrinsically linked with American corporatism. It isn't. And while some people can shout themselves hoarse blindly defending a subject that most of them likely haven't ever researched for themselves, you can rest assured that no big agribusiness is going to have your back, when your and your kids medical bills start building up.

Further, your average Americans diet is saturated in soy and high fructose corn syrup. This being the case, GMO is in nearly everything that we eat and drink in America, that comes either foil sealed, wrapped in plastic, or boxed in cardboard, in your local supermarket freezer section.

Anyone remotely concerned about their long term health, needs to therefore take a step back and say, "okay do I want to trust an industry which neither wants to label its produce or allow independent scientific analysis of its produce, in regard to it's long term effects on the human body?"

Besides, even without adding GMO's into the equation, you can put a chicken breast in between two slices of bread, and already you have arsenic, titanium oxide, your coal tar derived additives, and your brominated flour to worry about.

This being the case, I can hold my hands up and say, hey, maybe after five years of independent study and testing, GMO will actually turn out to be the best thing that humans have had arrive on their dinner table since bread and butter.

Right here and right now however, not only has that five years not happened yet, but I've already got enough to deal with, with the monosodium glutamate and the artificial sweeteners that the FDA told me were safe without actually testing.

Not to mention the stuff that's in what used to be my favorite brand of hot dogs, that they openly admit is going to make me fat and give me cancer.

Do I personally therefore want to to take a risk on including biotech produce in my diet? Nada.

Especially given that no one will let me know what happens if a rat eats it for more than thirty days.

~ It's Not The Freaking Wheat America ~

COULD IT REALLY BE SO EASY?

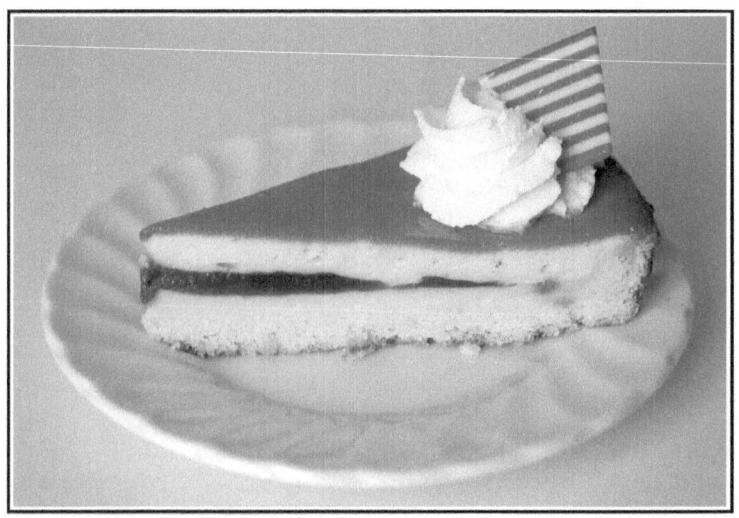

I know. You have spent so long being told that your present weight is down solely to your own level of inactivity and those unchangeable genes of yours, that it's difficult to come to terms with the fact that your size might not actually be your fault.[10]

However, for at least one demonstrable example of the provable relationship between consumption of GMO produce and obesity in particular, the graph

10 Image courtesy of Tim Nooteboom aka pr3vje at www.sxc.hu

on the next page has been sourced from a March 2013 Examiner article.

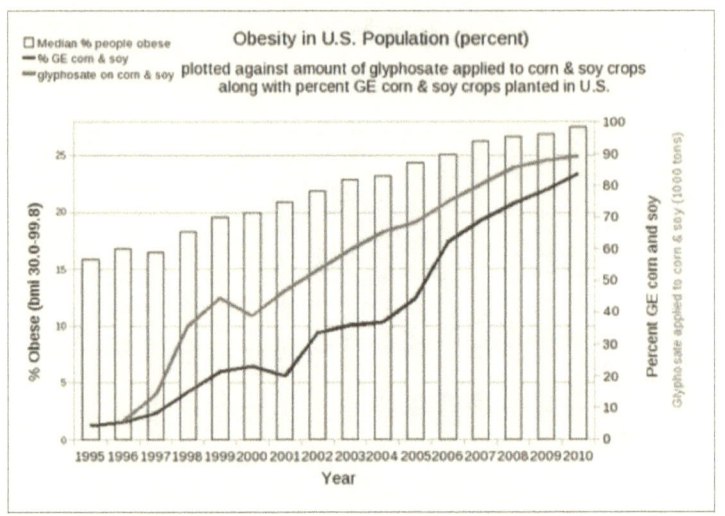

You see, what the above shows, is that in the 15 years between 1995 and 2010, (1994 being being the first year that GMO crops became permissible for sale in America) obesity in America almost doubled in parallel with both the amount of GMO's on the market and the amount of ghyphosate being used on GMO crops during cultivation in order to keep pests at bay.

But hey you know what? Don't just take my word on that.

Rather, here's something that you can do at home:

Go to your den, clear a space on the floor, get your family album out and line all the photos of yourself and your family side by side in order of when they were taken up until, and then after 1995.

You see, you can make this real (or not) for yourself, simply by looking back at your own photographs from the past twenty to twenty five years, and identifying for yourself which years have seen you struggle most with your weight.

In fact, you might find it worth your while to try and pinpoint when it was exactly, that you started having trouble with your weight in the first place.

You see, the simple fact of the matter, is that most people are going to see that they started having trouble with their weight in the mid to late nineties, and that despite all their best efforts since then they have probably only got bigger and more unhealthier looking.

What has also happened since the nineties however, is that American society seems to have been indoctrinated into the deranged belief that it's lower sex drive, weight gain, gastric discomfort, lethargy, diabetes, fertility problems and you name it, is all just something that happens to everyone as they get older.

Sorry to burst your bubble here though America, but come on, seriously?

You see, when I was a kid I don't remember people in their thirties and forties not being able to fit on a park bench comfortably. Yeah there was something called being fat, but specialist clothes stores catering for 'big and tall' people and digestive health clinics littered everywhere? I'm afraid not.

You know what though? Don't think that I'm getting all nostalgic on you here, get online and watch some old newsreels.

Make it an American practical history exercise for the whole family, and watch some old civil rights movement videos from the 60's and 70's, and keep an eye on the crowds as you do. Because you won't see many, if any people the size and shape that we are today.

In fact, it was the norm until the late eighties really, for most people to stay relatively trim until their mid fifties.

Besides, if it had always been the norm for us to be big by our thirties, have diabetes and IBS by the time we're 40, and for 34% of us to be pretty much physically disabled by our weight by the time that we're in our fifties, I'm sorry but America simply wouldn't have made it this far.

This is a new thing. Period.

Could however, it really be so simple to fix as you simply ditching the GMO, the additives, the artificial sweeteners and the refined sugar in your daily diet? Well hey, how about you tell me?

You see, I can sit here and talk and reel off numbers and throw the occasional chart at you. You however, are the only one who can put this to the test for yourself.

Moreover, and as I've already tried to assert, until you find your own rhythm in your own kitchen, this ain't easy.

The thing is though America, if you're anything more than ten or twenty pounds overweight, you need to put as much distance as possible, between you and the idea that it's ever going to be easy to loose what you want to loose in the time you want to loose it in.

There's never going to be a legitimate way for you to burn, shed, shred or juice your way to Skinnyville in the long term. Not unless you're prepared to pay for some kind of surgery.

You see, if there was, you wouldn't be paying $12.99 to Mr Just Juice Everything, and Mrs Get The Hell Away From The Bread Roll, for their new book every couple of months or so.

Rather, you'd be talking to your neighbor about

how effortlessly he or she lost two hundred pounds just by juicing or going on the Jared Fogle regimen, because after twenty years, the secrets of such a miraculous weight loss regimen, would have filtered through by now into becoming common knowledge already.

The reason then that such secrets haven't, is due simply to the fact that every so called solution out there is far from being viable in the long term.

Start juicing. Start looking and feeling fantastic. But now look at what you're doing. You're not sitting down for a meal with the person you love at the end of the day, and if you are you're feeling bad about it.

In fact, if you ask me, the idea of abiding to a permanent juicing regimen simply further deteriorates peoples already shaky psychological and emotional relationship with real food.

America doesn't need to be put on nil by mouth just so as to get healthy again. She needs a satisfying and sustainable in the long term life style choice.

This then is what I'm trying to give you. But I'm sorry America, I can't make twenty years of ugly go away in just one weekend.

Moreover, if you do take up this regimen you have

to do it properly.

You see, I've got a lot of friends who diet and almost all of them do something that I like to call pick and mix dieting. This being where they decide to follow a specific dietary regimen for a set length of time, but then in almost no time at all, deviate from that regimen because in part it's not 100% convenient to stick to it completely.

They don't trash their diet altogether. They just decide that they really need something that their diet seems to be diametrically opposed to, and so find some way to justify having that something anyway.

Let's say for example, that Joe America has decided to do the new Atkins diet and completely give up on carbs for a couple of weeks. The problem here is that Joe works in construction, has to take his lunch to work with him everyday, and thinks he's going to look kinda stupid just chewing on a pre-cooked beef steak come lunch time.

This being the case, Joe adapts his diet slightly in order to allow himself to have a single bread roll everyday.

Of course, that's a really oversimplified example, but hey, we've got vegetarians in America who somehow persuade themselves that it's still okay for them to eat chicken.

The point that I'm trying to make though, is that the 'cook for yourself' regimen which I'm trying to advocate, simply won't work for you if you try to cut corners. If therefore, you can't commit to the regimen completely, please don't try it.

Let's say for example, that you bake all your own bread, cook all your own meals, and even eat only 100% organic produce everyday. You see, although you might use all that to justify your allowance of a bottle of soda after lunch, as soon as that soda touches your lips you're ingesting brominated vegetable oil, coloring agents and quite possibly wood alcohol resembling artificial sweeteners, that by and large carry side effects which include obesity and diabetes.

In short, you're undermining the entire regimen by continuing to put something in your body which is inherently bad for you.

Likewise, if you decide that you simply don't have the time to bake your own bread, that's fine. Please be aware however, that shop bought bread is actually one of the main things which you should be avoiding.

You see, this isn't about cutting down on the amount of toxins you're exposing yourself to. Things like aspartame and monosodium glutamate don't work like calories, in that it's how much you have that matters. They work like drugs.

In fact, many people argue that many such additives actually are drugs. This being the case, using just one stock cube, having just one bottle of soda, and even though it sounds ridiculous, drinking just one glass of factory farmed milk, should be seen as equivocal to taking a pill every morning, that is designed to make the rest of what you eat ten times more toxic and fattening.

Some food additives after all, actually mimic hormones such as the female sex hormone estrogen. A fact which has been linked to both male breast development syndrome, (that a significant amount of overweight American males presently suffer from) fertility and sexual dysfunction problems, (in both men and women) and even cancer.

In the simplest of terms then, when you have a chemical or an additive like that, it doesn't matter whether you have half a teaspoon or a full two liter bottle.

It's not food. It's not going to be recognized by your body as food. It's not therefore going to be lifted out of your bloodstream by your organelles. Instead it's just going to keep on circulating in your bloodstream, triggering a range of hormonal and in many cases inflammatory bodily responses, until your liver can either figure out how to get rid of it.

101

(After identifying that it's not actually a real hormone). Or if it can't, simply store it safely encased in fat cells.

In fact, a great example to use here is the food additive olestra, an artificial fat substitute that a lot of chips are cooked in to reduce their overall calorie count.

You see, olestra passes into peoples blood streams through the gut, but is actually too big a molecule for peoples bodies to actually metabolize.

On paper then this sounds great, and anyone dieting might well be forgiven for thinking that they can still eat as many packets of chips or rice snacks as they like, because of how crazily low in calories they are.

Here's the kicker though, you see, a lot of vitamins and minerals are fat soluble, and are only processed by our body after being mixed with fats in our gut.

Olestra might therefore sound great, but what actually happens when people ingest it, is that although it captures the fat soluble vitamins waiting in the gut, and although it takes them into our bloodstream where they are needed, the organelles who's job it is look out for essential vitamins and minerals simply don't see them, because the olestra molecule itself is biochemically unprocurable.

This being the case, olestra effectively strips peoples bodies of essential vitamins, minerals, and even cancer and disease fighting plant pigmentation molecules called carotenoids.

So yeah, your chips and your spread might say they are fat free, but really they're the last things you want to be putting in your body or incorporating with any kind of diet, if you're really trying to loose weight.

In fact, by stripping your body of the nutrients it needs, you're in the very least case going to work up one hell of an appetite.

Further, lets look at milk and dairy. You see, from my experience I can tell you straight that these are the three main areas that people are either going to fail on, or in the least case try to cut corners.

Baking all your own bread is simply too inconvenient for most people. People by and large seem need something to snack on that they can't seem to make enough of themselves. And dairy? Well dairy gets expensive once you have to buy organic.

America's dairy industry however, has just as much to answer for as the FDA and America's GMO industry.

You see, in 1993, America's dairy industry began dosing its dairy herds with a bovine growth hormone, genetically engineered by one of America's leading agribusiness giants.

The problem however, with rBGH as it's known, is that although it forces cows to produce more milk than they normally would, it puts cows at much greater risk of developing udder infections. Something which in 79% of cows dosed with the drug, subsequently causes pus to be present in the milk milked from them.

Even worse, injecting cows with rBGH stimulates overproduction of another hormone called 1GF-1. One which regardless of species, works in all mammalian young to spur growth and in general development.

In both infant and adult humans however, the up to 5x increases in 1GF-1 is proven to disrupt normal cell division and in turn cause cancer.

Moreover, although pasteurization might kill bacteria from cow pus, 1GF-1 and the antibiotics that dairy cows are continually dosed with to keep their udder infections under control, easily out survive this process.

Quite literally then, every glass of milk that you drink is medicated. Further, 1GF-1 isn't just in your milk. It's in your cheese, your butter, your yogurt, many of your store bought baked goods, and even your milk chocolate.

I am not therefore saying that you have to do this regimen properly if you want to see results, just to cover my own back if you don't.

Rather if you simply can't cut out completely, the stuff that's making you fat and ill to start with, you are not going to see the results that you want.

This being the case, no, you loosing weight and taking back control over your health isn't going to be easy. You're going to have to use your loaf to figure out what's 100% safe to eat and what isn't. You're going to have to reorganize your finances so as to be able to buy what organic produce you need. You're going to have to bust a gut in the kitchen every day and hey, you're going to find that your relationship with family and friends is tested by you no longer grabbing a coffee together.

It is possible however, to overcome such challenges. All you need to ask yourself is, are you as committed and emotionally strong as you're going to need to be?

~ It's Not The Freaking Wheat America ~

DIETING THE DEADLY WAY

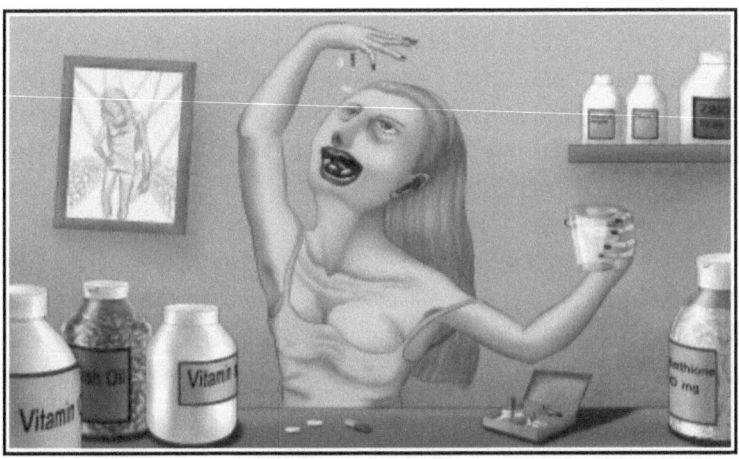

There are over one thousand reviews on Amazon for the diet pills I used to take. In fact when I think about it, I was pretty messed up a few years ago.[11]

I didn't like the way I looked, I didn't like the way that I felt physically in my own body, I was tortured by this feeling that I wasn't physically or intellectually interesting enough to ever have a successful long term relationship, and because of this feeling like the sum total of my overall spiritual identity, I was depressed.

---

11 Image courtesy of holohololand at FreeDigitalPhotos.net

Moreover, just like millions of Americans, I was willing to try anything to improve myself. Hence my arrival one day, at the online product review pages for different kinds of mail order diet pills.

Diet pills however, are one of America's dirty little dietary secrets, and I quickly found out why no one ever seems to want to talk openly about their latest experience with the latest fat burner nine thousands on the market.

It was 10am on a mid July morning in 2007. Two hours earlier, I'd taken two of the fat burners that had came in the mail the day before, and not thinking anything more about the matter I'd went on to get ready for work as normal.

Then, all of a sudden, BAM! The pills kicked in just as I was pulling out of my apartment parking lot.

Straight away I'd realized that I was in no fit state to drive, and it was nothing short of a miracle that I managed to re-park my car.

Somehow however, I did and a few minutes that felt like hours later, I was standing looking at myself in horror in the mirror in my apartment hallway.

I called my work. "S- S- Steven," I managed to speak into my phone. "I- I'm really really sorry....... b-bbut I'm not going to be able to make it in today." Then I hung up, and as I did I realized with an immediate sense of dread, that I'd just called in sick to work, without actually giving a reason.

I didn't trust myself enough however, to call my boss back and fake some kind of illness. I was high, and it was the most uncomfortable physical and psychological sensation that I'd ever experienced.

My heart was pounding. I felt cold and prickly all down my front. For some reason I felt like I should rush and do something, and looking at myself in the mirror, I knew that I couldn't let anyone see me while I was feeling like this.

One thing that wasn't so unpleasant however, was this sucked in feeling I had in my stomach.

Laying down on the sofa, I was then struck with the realization that what I'd actually done when I'd taken diet pills for the first time in my life that morning, was taken amphetamines.

Suddenly then, part of the world started to make sense to me.

You see, I'd never really got why celebrities are always found dead alongside concoctions of pills, or how these people you see on DR Phil, could go from being the kind of person you'd like to live next door to, to crystal meth addicts at the click of someone's fingers.

Suddenly however, all that made sense to me. You see, despite the uncomfortable-ness of the high itself, I was loving the stomach sucked in feeling.

In fact, in a bizarre way I already felt thinner after just one dose, and as mad as it might sound, I already knew that I was going to take some more the next morning, and perhaps even the next morning after that.

I thought therefore, of the crazy pressure that even the most fantastically wealthy celebrities must deal with everyday just to stay looking fantastic. Then I though of all those housewives who inexplicably start smoking crack, and in each case I could suddenly self identify with these people.

You see, although I couldn't possibly have magically just been made fifty pounds lighter, I both physically felt like I had, and I wasn't hungry. Slimmerville therefore, suddenly seemed not just nearer, but realistically achievable and affordable a place to start looking to move to in the long term.

All I'd need to do to get there and start living the ideal life I wanted, is find a way to manage this overbearing fuzzy feeling and I'd be fine. (Providing of course, that I didn't go crazy and start taking anything stronger.....).

Two weeks later and twelve pounds lighter however, my body hit some kind of barrier. Yeah I'd found a way to manage the high. In fact, I'd actually started to like having the extra energy. But after two weeks, not only was the weight not falling off as quickly as it has been, but I was starting to feel hungry again.

This being the case, and despite the fact that I was feeling like I'd been hit by a truck when I got up most mornings, I started to think about getting some stronger pills to tied me over until I'd lost a full forty pounds.

Moreover, I justified this by telling myself that as soon as I was a full forty pounds lighter, I'd have the confidence to join a gym or an exercise class, and loose the rest of the weight that I wanted to the old fashioned way.

Getting stronger pills, I then went through the whole 'Bam!' of feeling high and uncomfortably fidgety again. However, because I had expected it this time, I popped the first ones over the weekend, and by Monday morning felt confident enough to drive to work and function pretty much as well as I had learned to on my previous brand.

For all intensive purposes in fact, it took less than two weeks in 2007, to turn me into a diet pill junkie.
A month later however, I hit another barrier. You see, although by then I'd lost over twenty pounds, I realized that I was actually just maintaining the weight that I had got to, by using the pills as

111

appetite suppressants.

The barrier that I therefore found myself with my back against this time, was my own bathroom door as I realized that I was never really going to be able to stop taking the pills completely.

Once again however, I in the end justified this by mentally repeating to myself what it said on the pills product description. This being that they were made of 100% natural ingredients.

Of course, I did in the end stop taking them completely.

That November, a friend came right out and told me that everyone had noticed that I seemed wired all the time, and an overwhelming sense of shame and embarrassment subsequently saw me ditch what had by then become three different brands of miracle fat burners in the garbage.

The next day I then celebrated by ordering a bucket of chicken with extra fries and gravy from a place near by, before watching a marathon of back to back episodes of Lost.

The chicken, fries, and gravy however, were not the reason as to why by the middle of the next week, I'd put on nearly all the weight that I had lost. You see, what I came to realize quite quickly, was that the pills which I had been taking were for the most part diuretics. I had essentially therefore, been keeping myself in a state of permanent dehydration for over three months.

This then, was why I had been feeling like I didn't have the strength to get out of bed most mornings, and why at first the pounds had seemed to fall off me, just like all the reviews online said that they would.

What I further realized, was that for over three months I'd been a complete wreck. My work and social life had revolved exclusively around me continually trying to hide the fact that I was high. I hadn't been sleeping properly. I'd been paranoid. And remember that sucked in feeling which I thought felt so good in the beginning? Well, after three months and a few days off of my miracle elixir, I sat on my sofa with a hand on my stomach thinking, "Jesus, what the hell have I being doing to myself?"

If therefore, I come across sometimes as a little pushy when I say that you can't cheat if you do this, or a little too critical of other diet regimens out there, it's not because I'm small minded or bare some kind of grudge.

It's because I've been there. I've tried tens of diet regimens, I've popped the pills, I've applied the conductive jelly to the electric muscle pads they say that you work out with just by wearing, and I've even tried living off two turkey sandwiches a day from Subway.

Now however, diet books and infomercials saying that you're guaranteed to get in shape in no time if you just buy this, or throw some money at whatever new thermal corset, some world renowned fitness guru somewhere has invented, just makes me angry.

You see, there's a multi-million, perhaps even multi-billion industry out there that says it can fix your dissatisfaction with your size. Really though this industry is just outright dangerous.

Yeah, some might argue that I got what I deserved by trying diet pills. However, that doesn't change the fact that there are millions of American's out there similarly so desperate to loose weight that they are going to try them to.

People's weight depresses them. It gets some people so down that they take their own life because of it.

Knowing now then, that just eating properly is what people need to be doing to start looking better and feeling better about themselves, it disgusts me that there are some people out there who seem to be happy to capitalize on such misery.

There is for example, a diet book presently on the

market which documents one American woman's triple digit weight loss, which she achieved through pretty much just eating her favorite fast foods while counting the calories.

Moreover, yeah, the woman looks great compared to how she used to look when she weighed an extra 130 pounds. I personally however, can't think of anything more dangerous to say to a fat person.

You see, anyone can loose weight no matter what they eat if they count and accordingly restrict their calorie intake.

Further, with fast food being almost every modern Americans vice when it comes to how they maintain the XXL shirt sizes that they do, who isn't going to want to believe that they can get trim in no time by eating three square meals a day at their favorite burger bar?

I have not however, lied or spent my spare time simply making stuff up about what is really in most processed food, and pretty much every carton of fries that you will ever pick up.

Check everything that I've said so far out for yourself.

This being the case, it grates me to see someone openly encouraging people to ditch their vegetables in favor of topping themselves up everyday with toxic artificial flavor enhancers, indigestible coal and petroleum derived coloring agents, and hydrogenated trans-fats.

Hell, the woman might as well have titled her book: 'How To Loose Weight And Exponentially Increase Your Risk Of Having A Heart Attack And Getting Cancer.'

Similarly, a weight loss blog post which I read recently, detailed how for every kilogram of ice a person eats, they burn something like 200 calories just by trying to re-balance their bodies core temperature.

Sounds harmless and maybe even fun. Especially if you're an ice cream junkie. However, by lowering your bodies temperature, you're actually also lowering the pace at which enzymes and bacteria in your gut start digesting what foods already in there. Do I therefore think that that such a process is advisable? No.

In fact, there are a plethora of diet smoothie recipe books out there at present, which actually advise people to top up their fruit and yogurt smoothies, with sugar free shop bought deserts to add taste and texture.

Let's just be clear about this though, this means that somebody is advocating a seemingly super healthy diet, by them advising that you load yourself up on artificial sweeteners every day. Ones which are proven to spur the onset of numerous diseases and even contribute to weight gain and obesity.

Knowing what I know about food and nutrition, I therefore peruse such titles and blog posts in abject revulsion.

I mean don't get me wrong, I get it. Joe America who likes grabbing a McGriddle in the morning and stopping back off at the drive through after work to get a double quarter pounder or a box of popcorn chicken, simply wants to be told that he's allowed to eat what he wants when he wants it.

Then there's the trendy brigade who want to feel like they are part of the juicing and smoothie bandwagon, but still want to satisfy their sweet tooth somehow.

Regardless however, of whether there is a market for such materials, it abhors me to see what is essentially some of the most health detrimental advice anyone can ever possibly impart, routinely being sold as solutions to peoples pre-existing weight problems.

Moreover, don't get me wrong, calorie counting, juicing, loading yourself up with smoothies, doing the paleo diet, and following everything from the Atkins regimen, to the latest 5:2 diet will make you loose weight. Maybe that toning belt that you saw advertised recently will even tone your tummy up for you afterwards.

Besides, there will be people reading this who simply won't have the time to bake their own bread and wizz round town trying to find organic produce outlets in order to pick up some 1GF-1 free milk and yogurt. This being the case, and if weight loss is your one and only prerogative, dive into Amazon and find a book that outlines a diet regimen better suited to you individually.

As someone however, who wasn't happy with her weight for as long as they can remember, I haven't just embarked on a food journey in recent years that has seen me loose weight and feel comfortable finally in my own body. Rather, I've done something which has fundamentally reinvigorated me as a whole person.

You see, unlike on the diet pills that I experimented with in 2007, and unlike on calorie counting regimens and anti carb programs that I followed on and off for most of my adult life, I don't spend my life worrying about progress that I'm going to double back on if I decide to have a double helping of cheesecake after dinner every once in a while.

I don't feel psychically restrained in anyway in regard to what I am or what I'm not allowed to eat at any given moment. And I certainly don't find myself curling up into a ball some mornings, so loathing of my own body sense and reflection, that I don't want to get out of bed.

Moreover, I genuinely don't worry about falling sick with the same cancer or heart aliments which stole my father away in his fifties. Hell, I'm even more empowered politically than I was before.

I have not therefore, spent this book so far trying to scaremonger people in regard to what they are putting in front of their kids after school. Or for that matter, simply trash the work of professional dietitians and nutritionists who really do believe that one way or the other is the answer to better physical vitality.

Rather, I'm just trying to advocate a sustainable lifestyle choice that not just works, but one which genuinely puts you back in control of your own life and puts you on a path to becoming the person that you have always wanted to realize yourself as.

In fact, late last year I was serving up pot roasted crispy butter chicken breasts, sautéed baby potatoes, peas and a creamy mushroom sauce that I had decided to experiment in making; and as I got the table ready I was talking the ears off my hubby, in regard to how there are a catalog of mushroom varieties that I'm still dying to get my hands on.

Then, as we sat down to eat, my other half said

119

"Chelsea, you know I never really thought about it ever before, but you're exactly the woman I always pictured myself raising a family with."

And you know what? Although we haven't decided to do that just yet, I felt in that moment that I'd finally become the woman who I'd always wanted to be. An educated, happy in her work, home, and mind and body woman, who even though she's far from materially wealthy, has exactly what she's always wanted.

You see, food isn't just something that you eat to satisfy your hunger. The more wholesome what you eat is, the more wholesome a whole person you are.

EXPENSE AND PRACTICALITY

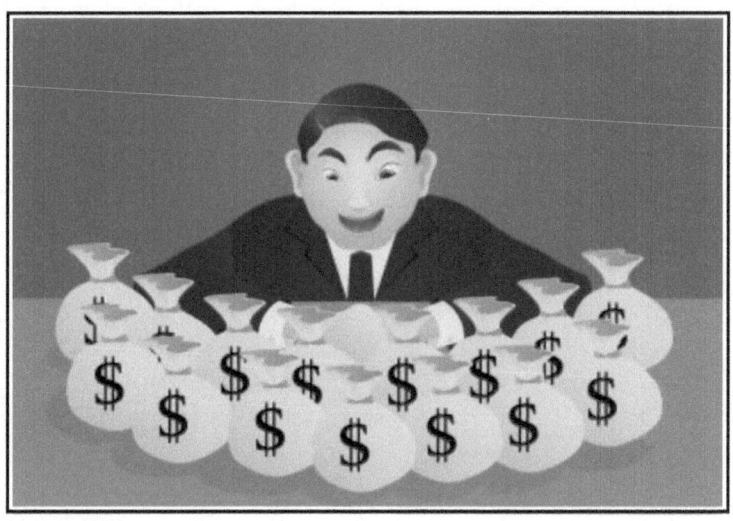

Okay. I get it. One, you already can't see how you could incorporate such a regimen into your daily and weekly life because of time concerns. Two, organic produce in America tends to cost between 20% and 100% more than what most people are used to picking up in their local Walmart. And three, a lot of people reading this won't just have themselves to think about, many people will have families and young children.[12]

---

12   Image courtesy of holohololand at FreeDigitalPhotos.net

Now I'm not going to try and belittle peoples monetary concerns. I know what it's like to sign up to a new diet regimen and experience that sinking feeling, as soon as you realize that there's simply no way that you will be able to afford half of the fresh produce that you need.

As for time however, you do have it, you probably just don't know it yet. Everyone has at least a day or two off work each week (if not you seriously need to think about looking for a better job) and one day if you set your mind to it, is all you really need to set you up for most of the next week.

This meaning get most, (if not all) of your baking done, and if need be prepare in advance your entire week to comes evening meals.

Just make sure to run to the grocery store the afternoon or evening after work the day before, so as to stock up on everything you're going to need ingredients wise.

Here in fact, is why it's so important to make a list of your favorite meals.

You see, prior to going to the store you are going to have to look at that list and subdivide each meal into a list of the consecutive ingredients that you are going to need to make it.

Let's say for example, that you have Spaghetti

Carbonara on your list. First you would just write it down off the top of your head because you like it. (Along your other twenty or so meal ideas). Then, when the list is finished, you would go back to Spaghetti Carbonara, do a quick search on the Internet for the basic recipe, and from that be able to determine that to make it yourself, you are going to need spaghetti, bacon, black pepper, eggs and cheese.

In fact, what I used to do in the beginning, is copy and paste the basic recipe that I'd found, onto a document on my computer, and save it in a folder called recipes. This way, when I finally got around to making whatever I was making, I wouldn't get confused by any other recipes.

Moreover, always make sure to find the most basic recipes available. You're probably a novice in the kitchen, even if you don't think that you are, so be kind to yourself.

Now, with the ingredients that we have listed, i.e. bacon, cheese, black pepper, eggs, we need to sort these out into what needs to be bought organically in order to avoid GMO and additive contamination, and in this case that's everything apart from the black pepper.

For me personally though, I simply can't afford organic meats most of the time, therefore what I do is look first for grass fed conventional meats, and rather than buy things like bacon or ham, I will as I mentioned at the beginning, buy a whole joint of pork.

Not only is this usually cheaper, but if you pick up a packet of sliced bacon, turning that packet over you will usually find that it's swimming in additives to make it look pretty.

Now, once you have your list ready and have subdivided each meal into its respective ingredients, make sure also that you have included the ingredients for any baked goods like bread and pastry that you might need to make.

Moreover, although this sounds like a hassle it's really not. Besides, you might even be surprised by how much money you save when you have ordered your shopping list in such a way, and subsequently end up leaving your local grocery store minus any last minute purchases of whatever frozen pizzas were on offer this week.

However, what you also do when you order in such a way, is steadily start building up your very own recipe book. This being the case, although for the first couple of weeks you're still going to feel a little lost, a month or two from now you will have at least twenty tried and tested recipes that you know that you're fully capable of preparing.

Now, if you have a family, I would advise that you

try and find a way to adjust everyone in your households diet along with your own. Yes, this might cause arguments and hey, for all I know this might not actually be possible to accomplish given your specific situation.

However, here's the thing. When I mentioned earlier that preparing and cooking all your own food in this way completely changes your personal emotional relationship with food, I wasn't just talking about just you on an individual basis.

You see, we fall over each other and we bicker about it sometimes, but shortly after we moved in together, me and my other half quickly got into the routine of cooking and baking together as a team. I showed him how to make bread, and to my surprise, (and if I'm honest quiet jealousy) he turned out to be better at baking it than me.

This being the case, my hubby is usually in charge of baking bread most of the time, whilst I rustle up everything from meatloaf to Moroccan lamb tagine, croissants, and even cheesecake.

Moreover, when we do have children, it's going to be both our priorities in terms of their education and health, for us to introduce them to wholesome food preparation as soon as possible.

You see, this is what family life used to be like in America. Kids helped with kneading dough and baking cookies, men worked to be able to put food on the table, and rather than being just a stereotypical housewife, a woman was the beating heart and the seat of the soul of the family.

Times have of course changed, but what we have found, is that if both me and my hubby participate equally in preparing our food for the week ahead, we both become the spiritual center of our family, and this is what food should be for everyone. A family experience that everyone is involved in to some degree.

Food should never be an American mum calling her overweight kids out from the den when a microwave ping's. Nor should a families experience of eating together be one where they simply unbox burgers and spill fries out of cartons, before jumping back in the car and going home to their separate lives in front of separate computer screens.

Besides, by involving your family in your new dietary regimen, you're educating them as to why wholesome food is essential for their own health and nutrition.

Moreover, that isn't just something that's going to stick in their heads for the length of their childhood. Rather, that's the kind of education that they are likely going to impart to their own family one day too.

As such, you're not just teaching your own kids about how to eat healthy, you're quite possibly teaching your future grandchildren and perhaps even their grandchildren after them.

Of course, I haven't had children yet. This being the case, anyone reading this could perhaps accuse me of being over idealistic. I can assure you however, that this is only because I don't yet have the practical experience of getting up in the night and doing the school run.

One thing is for certain though, and that is that no child of mine will ever associate a rewarded for good behavior or family celebrations such as birthdays, with trips to their favorite fast food restaurant. Neither will they ever be encouraged to associate satisfying their hunger with a reach to a cupboard full of chips and candy.

In fact, by fifth grade any son or daughter of mine, is going to to know how to make everything from soda bread to home made pasta and a basic pot roast.

Furthermore, they are going to be fully educated by that time, in regard to what things like aspartame are proven to do to their bodies, and why it's in their own best interest to stick with a slice of home baked Mississippi mud cake if they want a treat, rather than a trip to the nearest candy store.

There is the chance of course, that you for whatever reason either don't want to, or simply can't involve your whole family in your new regimen and that's fine.

From a practical standpoint however, that will test you, and as I've said previously, if short term weight loss is your prerogative, maybe think about trying a different diet regimen, whilst perhaps building slowly towards this one.

Moreover, having your partner and your wider family involved in helping you in the kitchen, even if it's just to the extent of helping clean the dishes, makes cooking and baking all your own food feel a hundred times easier.

To get back on track however, let's assume that you have your twenty meal ideas listed, you have a basic recipe for each, and you have subdivided each meal into its consecutive ingredients.

Let's assume further, that you have done all the grocery shopping that you need to, and that like I suggested, you have decided to cook up a pot of broth to last you for a couple of days or more as you get to work baking.

You see, cooking a pot of broth or goulash, really helps put your mind at ease. It's there, it's easy to prepare, and even if everything goes wrong during your first baking experiences, you have already got your first wholesome home made food already prepared and steaming away on the counter.

Now, to make things easier in regard to making bread, use the most basic recipe you can find which requires yeast, and even if that recipe is for a loaf of bread, try first to make buns.

Buns are easier to portion than a loaf of bread, and if you burn a loaf you usually burn it all. Whereas with buns you don't usually burn the whole batch, and buns are by and large more versatile than a whole loaf.

In fact, it's far easier to plan ahead with buns.

Looking to bake 20, for example, gives you a sandwich for lunch every day, buns for burgers one evening and 11 extra for whenever you feel like having a sandwich for a snack or toasting half for supper.

The trickiest part of baking bread however, is getting it to rise and this is where most people loose faith in their own potential as a self taught baker.

What I have found however, is that using a splash of warm milk to activate whatever yeast you decide to use, before kneading the dough consistently for twenty minutes, usually brings my bread up perfectly.

To knead, make sure that your dough is loose and pliable but not sticky, and then push the fingers of both your hands into it, before withdrawing them and immediately folding the dough over itself. Kneading and folding like this will trap the air in the dough to make it lighter, and in repeating this process for twenty minutes or more, the warmth of your own hands will itself work to start the yeast working.

In regard then to setting your dough aside to rise, I have a closet which I put a small oil heater in on low, and leave my dough to rise in there, as I've never been able to successfully get it to rise over my cooker. The key seems to be to keep it covered and exposed to a consistent temperature of around eighty six degrees.

Also if you mess up don't throw anything away! I burnt bread and I made the equivalent of baked meteorites when I started baking, and stupidly I threw away my failed batches.

As it is however, when you make meatballs or meatloaf, you can actually double the volume of mince meat that you have, by grating into crumbs and mixing in even the stalest and most disastrous of your failed bread experiments.

In fact, processed food manufacturers pad mechanically rendered meat out in exactly the same way, only they use soy protein.

Moreover, I always make sure to bake a little extra bread, as you can use grated bread crumbs to bread fish and meat, and even veggie burgers. Not to mention fry up pieces of stale bread with olive oil and garlic to make scrumptious soup croûtons.

Now, because I usually give my bread two to three hours to rise, I use that time to cook up sauces. I usually make around a liter of cheese sauce and a liter of tomato and basil. This way I can decide last minute at any time through the week, to cook up carbonara, bolognaise, lasagna, cauliflower cheese and various other pasta and baked vegetable dishes.

Usually, I will then put these in a couple of containers in the fridge, clean up, put my bread in to bake, and then spend the latter half of the day baking a range of savories and deserts.

Often I'll bake cheese spinach and bacon quiche, some spicy vegetable and lentil samosas for snacks, and then finish off with a tray of gingersnaps made using real grated root ginger.

Of course, what I make varies, but this is the general gist of my average Saturday.

Now, look at what I have. I have vegetable and chicken broth for at least two days, bread for at least a week, sauces preprepared so that all I have to do if I want, is boil up some pasta after getting in late from work, a quiche that makes a great alternative to taking sandwiches to work, samosas to snack on, and even ginger snaps.

In fact, I always finish the week with a surplus of food. Moreover, once you develop a routine like this you realize that sticking to a regimen such as this one isn't actually expensive or overly time consuming.

Because I'm not picking up a sub at lunch time, a coffee on the way to work, or a box of chicken on the way home, I'm actually saving at least $3-$4 dollars a day, which more than covers the increased cost of staples like pasta and dairy produce that I insist on buying organically.

Similarly, because I've organized my shopping list so consciously, I'm in and out of the store in record time each week. And even then I notice that I'm actually saving more money than I used to on my groceries.

Further, because I've often got most of my meal preparation for any night of the week done already, I actually find that I have extra time after work each evening just to unwind.

Honestly then, the only initial pitfalls of this regimen are the ones that are in your own mind. Yes, you have to deal with temptation just like you have to do on every diet regimen. However, rather than fret over what you think you are and are not capable of, and what you can and can't afford, you just have to motivate yourself to plan and try it out for yourself.

I will bet however, that there are now some food and health fanatics decrying the fact that I am not insisting that everyone buy all organic when it comes to their weekly grocery run.

In fact, I'll bet that there is a dietitian out there banging his or her head now, in abject horror at the amount of wheat that I've included in my regimen.

Here's the thing though, I simply can't afford to buy all organic. I would if I could but I can't.

If one week I have a significant surplus of food in the fridge, I'll make sure to spend what I would normally spend on food anyway, and treat myself to organic meat.

Moreover, I know that ideally everyone should be eating organically. I know that pesticides and herbicides like glyphosate are bio-accumalative and show up in 90% of peoples urine as far away as the Mediterranean.

I can not change the fact however, that at present I can't afford to go organic full time.

If however, you can afford to go organic, do it. Not just because the produce that you will be eating will be healthier and more nutritious, but because for more of a demand for organic produce, the more land will eventually be turned over for organic cultivation.

More organic farming jobs will then be created, and because supermarket chains will see that it's profitable to invest in, and source produce from America's organic farms, the price for such produce will eventually become relative for people like me, and most other Americans to realistically afford.

As for the wheat deal, you can still do this regimen if you have been convinced already that you should ditch the wheat in order to ditch your bulging bits. All you have to do is substitute organic wheat flour for organic spelt flour or some other grain.

In fact, I use spelt occasionally for making pancakes.

Personally however, not only does it trouble me how seemingly esteemed nutritionists and scientists can decry wheat itself as having caused America's obesity crisis, whilst somehow omitting to mention the shoe rubber and the coal tar, but also, I simply prefer wheat bread and I've still managed to get healthy.

Lastly, for anyone who is still undecided and perhaps even thinks this is all silly, I went to the store this afternoon and bought a preprepared quiche advertised as low in calories and as containing no artificial ingredients.

You see, I've been in stores with my friends and even my partner when we first met, and knowing me they always seem to want to make a fuss over the fact that they are picking this brand or that brand because it's 100% natural and low fat and the like.

Here however, is the list of ingredients for this 100% natural product:

Filling:
Milk, Swiss Cheese (Part Skim Milk, Cheese Cultures, Salt, Enzymes), Eggs, Water, Cooked Bacon ([Cured With Water, Salt, Sugar, Sodium Phosphates, Sodium Erythorbate, Sodium Nitrite], Smoke Flavor, Dextrose, Potassium Chloride), Cornstarch, Onions, Whey Protein Concentrate (Milk), Seasoning (Salt, Spices), Chives.

Pastry:

Enriched Flour (Wheat Flour, Niacin, Iron, Thiamine Mononitrate, Riboflavin, Folic Acid), Butter (Cream, Salt), Water, Canola Oil, Salt, Soy Lecithin. Contains Eggs, Milk, Soybeans, Wheat,

Florentine Filling: Milk, Eggs, Swiss Cheese (Part Skim Milk, Cheese Cultures, Salt, Enzymes), Spinach, Cornstarch, Water, Onions, Whey Protein Concentrate (Milk), Chives, Onions, Salt (Contains Soybean Oil), Nutmeg, Flack Pepper. Pastry: Enriched Flour (Wheat Flour, Niacin, Iron, Thiamine Mononitrate, Riboflavin, Folic Acid), Butter (Cream, Salt), Water, Canola Oil, Salt, Soy Lecithin. Contains Eggs, Milk, Soybeans, Wheat.

You see, it's very likely that the soy and the cornstarch here is genetically modified. The thing is though, because of anti-GMO labeling laws lobbied for by the industry itself, you're not allowed to know either way.

Even however, if they're not, we still have the cancer causing, but good for aesthetic purposes sodium nitrate hitching a ride along with the bacon. Not to mention sodium phosphate that is proven to cause kidney damage.

What worries me the most about this product however, is the fact that I happen to make Quiche Lorraine quite a lot, and I can't for the life of me understand why there is soybean oil, canola oil, soybeans themselves or things like cornstarch in here in the first place.

Quiche Lorraine is cheddar cheese, bacon, tomatoes, thyme, eggs, milk, cream and salt and pepper and that's it.

The only reason I can think of as to why anyone would have to put so much more in there, is if none of the above nine ingredients were of anywhere near decent quality........Or you were intentionally trying to poison someone.

And hey, that might sound overly dramatic, but at least start reading and cross referencing the freaking packaging on this stuff will you America?

IS SOMEONE INTENTIONALLY POISONING YOU?

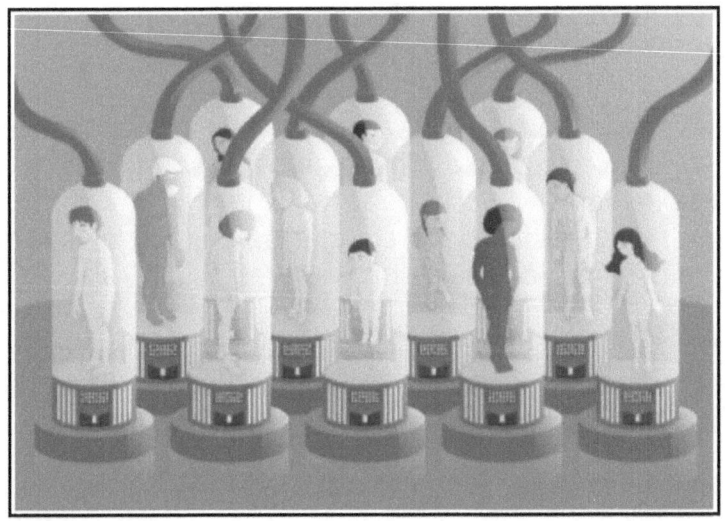

When we lost my father in 1995, I blamed the two people who I was then closest to, him and the Marlboro cowboy.[13]

As far as I was concerned, my dad hadn't ate well and he'd known it.

When we were kids he'd have cereal or sometimes

---

13 Image courtesy of holohololand at FreeDigitalPhotos.net

bacon biscuits and gravy for breakfast with me and my brother and sister every morning. But then an hour later he'd be in a diner down the road having sausage slices, bacon, eggs, and potato chips.

Most of the day to come, you'd then be hard pressed to find a single moment, when he didn't have a cigarette in his mouth.

In fact, even when he got diagnosed with cancer that the doctor told him straight was only going to be exasperated if he kept on smoking, my fathers first reaction had been to light up and bat away the idea like such an assertion was just silly.

Then, a year after my father passed, a man called Jeffrey Wigand came into my life. Jeffrey however, didn't arrive physically or even emotionally.

Rather, Jeffrey came into my life in the two dimensional sense, trapped behind the pixels of the cable television set in the den of what was still our family home in Perryville.

Jeffrey you see, told me and the world via CBS, that contrary to what they had been saying publicly for over fifty years, all the chief executives of all America's big tobacco companies, had known all along that nicotine in cigarettes was addictive, and that smoking itself causes cancer.

The tobacco industry he said, had even developed a

way of adding ammonia to tobacco, in order to make nicotine even more addictive. This despite the fact that the chemicals used in this process were known lung tissue carcinogens.

In no uncertain terms then, big tobacco had not just lied about whether nicotine was addictive. Rather, the tobacco industry had intentionally and premeditatedly researched and employed ways to make it even more addictive; knowing in the meanwhile that doing so would make many tobacco smokers terminally ill.

Unlike the rest of America however, I wasn't shocked by the fact that suddenly cigarettes were revealed as being addictive or carcinogenic.

I'd seen my father almost tear his own hair out, when on occasion he'd chanced to leave a carton at his work.

Moreover, I smoked and I knew fine well that it was more than just some kind of habit. Habits are things like flossing and curling your fingers through your hair absent mindedly. Neither of which makes your chest ache, or causes you feel physically irritable if you are ever prevented from doing them for some reason.

What did shock me though, was how stupid 99.9% of America turned out to be immediately after. You see, for years there had been this running debate as to whether cigarettes were addictive or health compromising.

Hell, up until 1995, some industry lobbyists were still trying to argue that although smoking wasn't good for you, there wasn't any verifiable proof that it was bad either.

In fact, scratch that. What shocked me after Jeffrey Wigand's appearance on 60 minutes in 1996, was how stupid 99.9% of the whole world subsequently came across as.

You see, I found myself sitting there a week later reading about class action lawsuits being filed, and I thought to myself, are these people serious?

I mean was America and the world really trying to tell me that no single government had had the real low down on how dangerous cigarettes were prior to Jeffrey Wigand?

That no single independent doctor or scientist had analyzed a packet previously and said, *"mmmhhh.... I'm starting to think that breathing in road tar laced with exotic ammonium compounds might not actually be all that sensible."*

I mean come on America, you went to the moon, you invented nuclear fission, and even by 1995 you were a wizz on computers. Are you seriously telling me that no one before 1996, had the faintest idea that nicotine was addictive, or that some, if not all cigarette ingredients were carcinogenic?

Of course they did.

Hence why after Wigand's 60 minutes interview, watching western countries reform their public health policies was like watching dominoes fall. No one could do it quick enough. And Why? Because every politician out there who had ever had any kind of affiliation with big tobacco, (which was all of them) was terrified of being called out publicly as a murderous crook.

Yet most Americans and most people around the world seemed not to be able to put two and two together, and realize that their respective government representatives and tobacco industries, had all been in on the deception.

You see, the reason that big tobacco got away with it for so long, is because it managed to lobby senior people affiliated with the FDA, in order to ensure that it (big tobacco) would be permitted do all its own product testing.

Similarly, big tobacco lobbied and petitioned politicians all over the world, in order to have international restrictions on cigarette sales and advertising relaxed significantly.

Hence why kids thought it was cool for a long while

to carry around candy cigarettes, and why my brothers toy racing cars always carried the same big tobacco painted on advertising slogans as their real life counterparts.

This being the case, I wasn't angry at my dad for very long after his passing. You see, he'd grown up in a world where because you can get away with anything if you have enough money, smoking itself had for the best part of his life actually been glamorized by American society.

Moreover, yes at some point it was my father who made a personal decision to smoke. However, not only did the people selling my father cigarettes flatly deny that they were remotely dangerous or addictive. But rather, over the course of the fifty years that my father smoked, these people actually researched and developed ways to purposefully make their products even more deadly.

It wasn't however, big tobacco who killed my father. Rather, it was over half a century of spineless and morally derelict men and women sitting in congress who stole my dad away.

In pursuit of their own wealth and social elevation, such people had after all, given big tobacco free license in the first place to lie, cheat, poison, and ultimately murder millions of American men and women. And this is something that we keep in mind when looking at the present state of America's food supply.

You see, politics in America at present, is just as inextricably linked with America's food industry as it once was with big tobacco.

Indeed, in United States diplomatic cables leaked by Wikileaks in 2011, no less than 926 of these documents discussed a U.S. government objective to promote the interests of private US biotechnology corporations, not just domestically, but around the world via the U.S. State Department.

US diplomats are detailed from 2005 in fact, as having been mandated to liaise with regional scientists, farmers and government representatives around the world in order to:

- Promote Biotech Business Interests
- Lobby Foreign Governments To Weaken Biotechnology Rules
- Protect US Biotech Exports
  And:
- Reach Out To The Developing World To Adopt Biotech Crop Strains

Further, the U.S. government is detailed at the same time, as having actively attempted to dissuade governments from around the world, from implementing so much as GMO labeling practices.

Put as simply as possible, billions of American tax dollars have been used since 2005, in order to lobby foreign governments on behalf of some of America's wealthiest corporations.

In fact, the parallels between what is presently happening with GMO and the relationship between the big tobacco and the American government for the most part of the last century are staggering.

Producers of GMO produce have lobbied the FDA in exactly the same way that big tobacco did, in order to be allowed to be solely responsible for vetting their own products safety.

Likewise, whereas big tobacco went around the world persuading governments to relax tobacco advertising regulations, GMO companies (being aware that in places like Europe, most people are fundamentally opposed to GMO produce) have simply lobbied against their products being advertised or even so much as labeled in the first instance.

Further, and just like big tobacco prior to Jeffrey Wigand, any scientist, agency, or public health group whom dares to say anything disparaging against GMO, is swiftly restrained by powers rising to the highest offices of American politics.

When for instance, British based scientist Arpad Pusztai, revealed on British television, the damning results of his own research into the effects of GMO consumption on rodents, it was a telephone call from then U.S. president Bill Clinton, to then British Prime Minister Tony Blair, which within twenty four hours saw Pusztai fired and legally gagged from further discussing his then research findings.

In short therefore, the very same tactics that big tobacco used to knowingly poison millions if not billions of people around the world for the best part of a century, are presently being employed by America's food industry.

More than that however, the very same U.S. agencies which facilitated big tobaccos premeditated poisoning of America, are once again facilitating the same, through their being so open (as always) to corporate lobbying.

Of Course, Congress and the FDA attempt to justify such lobbying, on the basis that less regulation of Americans food industry creates a better climate for big business to operate in.

However, it's not just America's food industry which benefits from such devil may care oversight.

Rather, for every American made sick from guzzling their artificial sweeteners and eating their cherished 'all natural' processed junk food and GMO, big pharma's waiting in the wings, just dying to get hold of your health insurance details.

Let's say for example, that you're one of those people who buys those make it yourself kits for pizza and cheesecake and chocolate muffins and the like.

Further, let's say that you picked up a make it yourself pepperoni pizza kit this afternoon, and that you plan on making it with your kids, so as to inject some fun into making dinner together.

You see, aside from the sodium nitrate and the soy and the cornstarch that we have already talked about at length, and aside from a few wacky things like cottonseed oil that you will find in such products; these bake it yourself kits often contain something which quite possibly comes near the top of the list of the most deadly things that you could ever want to find a reason to put into your body. This being sodium aluminum. Phosphate.

You see, aluminum. simply doesn't have any place in the human food chain. The food industry likes it though, as it makes things look white and it can act as a good emulsifier.

Things like bread, baking soda, cheese, confectionery, and pretty much anything else processed, is therefore literally full of the stuff.

People's bodies however, can neither metabolize or get rid of aluminum. once it has entered their digestive systems. This being the case, it accumulates slowly in people's bones and in significant amounts in people's brains, where it is proven after prolonged exposure, to cause things like Alzheimer's disease.

Coincidentally then, rates of Alzheimer's disease in the West, (just like cancer, autism, obesity and a host of other conditions) have dramatically increased in recent years. To the point where one in five Americans are presently advised that they are likely to develop the condition.

Of course, big pharma and even America's Alzheimer's Association don't seem to want to put two and two together publicly yet, and say "hey, "since we know that Alzheimer's is at least in part caused by aluminum. toxicity in the human body, shouldn't we perhaps stop putting it in the food that America's currently consuming?"

I mean why should they? Congresses February 2014 Alzheimer's Accountability Act now means that leading health industry experts on Alzheimer's disease, can every year until 2025, submit an annual budget to Congress asking for however much money they want in order to carry out research into the condition.

No one is therefore going to turn around tomorrow and say "hey, actually we figured it out already," and miss out on eleven years of un-capable funding.

Moreover, if no amount of experts could agree prior to 1996 that smoking cigarettes might be linked to conditions such as cancer, emphysema and heart disease, I personally don't put too much faith in this new bunch finding a cure for Alzheimer's just yet. Especially given the fact that the FDA and even America's State Department, are presently so cozy with America's corporate food industry.

As hard therefore, as it will be for most Americans to swallow, I'm afraid that someone is intentionally poisoning you.

Why? Well that bits the easy part. You see, you sitting down to have a 100% beef burger in a 100% real bread bun with 100% real potato fries just isn't profitable for middle men like America's agrochemical giants.

Hell, that way the money you spend on that meal only goes to the person who cooked it for you and the person who grew and produced the produce in the first place.

What America's middle men do therefore, is buy up all the beef, potatoes, and wheat grains, before cutting those ingredients like Columbian drug dealers, in order to make them go further.

You see, with the help of some dirt cheap soy and corn starch, they can make 5 burgers the same shape and size as the one you had before, and subsequently make five times as much profit as the original would make, at near the exact same cost price.

The only problem however, is that with all that padding it simply won't taste the same. This being the case, in goes some MSG and some other chemical flavorings, as well as some preservatives, and some things to make your nutritionally watered down burger look just as good, and hey presto, as far as you, the end consumer is concerned, nothing ever changed.

Yes, watching from the side lines big pharma might see that some people are starting to get sick, because what America is actually eating is nutritionally dead and by and large altogether toxic. But hey, for every public health concern that might come about, they're the ones charged with finding a cure.

Really, it's that simple. Further, don't be fooled when you see, lots of vitamins and minerals listed as added ingredients to your favorite brand of ready meal.

They are only there to compensate for the fact that they either don't occur naturally in the meal which you're about to eat, or more fiendishly, because something like olestra used to make it look and taste nice, is actually going to strip you of the vitamins and minerals already in your own body.

Of course, if you've read this book so far from the mindset of someone who only thinks in terms of how many calories they have per day, or how many carbs they have compared to how much protein they consume, you likely simply won't be able to grasp what it is that I am trying to relate to you here.

You see, most people categorize food as calories, fat, saturated fat, protein and carbohydrates and that's it. Me waltzing around saying "hey watch for the arsenic and the aluminum., and by the way America, this is probably why you presently look like some kind of beached sea creature," just sounds wacky to most people.

You owe it to yourself however, to at least start reading the packaging that your food comes in, and in turn ask yourself whether you want to continue putting products in your body, which to be honest you probably can't even pronounce the name of.

Moreover, with the precedent that the FDA and the tobacco industry set us in 1996, it's outright madness to assume that you can safely outsource your and your families nutritional well being, to the exact same kind of unquestionable corporatists.

And hey, yeah this might all sound crazy right now, but you know what? If you'd walked up to my father in 1965 and said, "hey Steve, you realize that those cigarettes are going to kill you one day don't you?" He would have likely just looked up from his pit in the garage and said something like, "you got a car needs fixin Mr? Or are you just here to throw around wild accusations?"

Unlike my late father however, our generation is more intellectually and technologically equipped to make informed decisions for itself, than any other that has ever came before it.

Hell, all people need to do before they put their favorite brand of chips in their shopping cart, is take out their smart phone and run an Internet search on each of the listed ingredients.

Do yourself a favor then America, and rather than take my word for anything that I have written here, go do your own research. Educate yourself, and once you have, start thinking about how you want to live the rest of your life and what you want to do about the fact that really your problem isn't that you need to loose weight.

Rather, it's that the folds, blotches, erupted blood vessels and in general unhealthy pallor of your full length reflection, is attributable solely to the fact that you've been steadily poisoned for most of your life, in the name of profit and convenience.

~ It's Not The Freaking Wheat America ~

PRACTICE CHILDREN

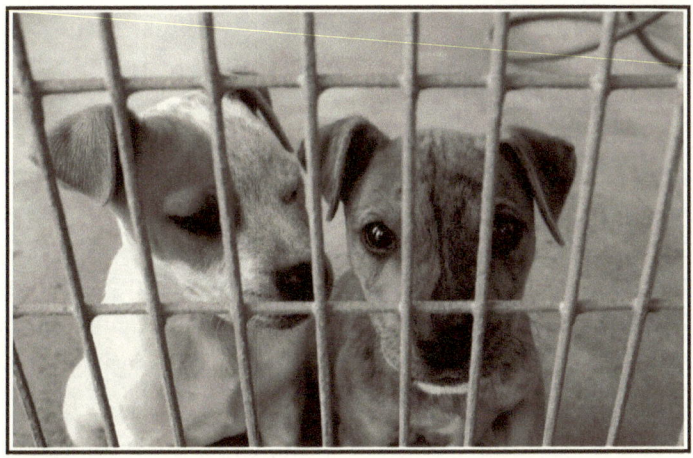

The chihuahua in the shelter had scars all over his body, a gaping open wound on his right back leg, was blind in one eye, and was obviously terrified of human beings. Further, although he was obviously in significant pain, he pinned itself regardless, into the furthest corner of his concrete cell, constantly cowering from the bark of the larger and much bolder animals penned either side of him.[14]

This being the case, the shelter person showing us around seemed to think that he was a lost cause

---

14 IMAGE COURTESY OF VEE BEE AKA ACADMEIC AT WWW.SXC.HU

and so strolled right past him at first. Even though me and Gary, (my then partner) had asked specifically to look at any small breeds they might have.

Deciding to ask about him myself, we were then told that he was brought in a few days earlier and that the shelter was pretty certain that he had been on the streets all his life.

Being about seven years old, not house trained and obviously in need of prolonged veterinary attention, the shelter didn't therefore see him as realistically adoptable. "Besides," he said. "Chihuahuas are classed by many people as toy dogs, and this one looks like it's just been in a car wreck."

It was only however, when the attendant mentioned prolonged veterinary care, that me and Gary looked at each other knowingly. We were after all, already planning to charitably adopt an old dog from a shelter rather than get a new pup, and it would be crazy to get one with an extra price tag attached.

As such, we moved on and were shown another Chihuahua in much better shape. One that was all wags and smiles and frantic bounds around as it realized that it was about to receive some human affection.

A little further along, we were then introduced to a still puppy terrier who was adorable to the extreme, and after him a boxer who though shy, still wagged her tail and bored her eyes into us longingly.

In fact, it was the boxer who got my then partner Gary excited. "Do you know how much a pedigree would cost?" He asked. "Plus she's a bitch."

I however, was still drawn to the chihuahua I'd asked about. Besides, a boxer was a bit bigger than what we had originally planned upon. Outside in the car, I therefore structured an argument along the lines of:

- The other dogs in the shelter obviously had much better chances of being adopted, and as such it would be more noble for us take him on, even if he was going to be a challenge.
- We could get a dog in perfect health and still find ourselves burdened by health problems.
- What kind of people were we if we adopted a dog just because of its looks, or the convenience of it already being trained? We were after all, looking to adopt as a kind of test to see what we might be like as parents.

Gary however, didn't take kindly to the suggestion that he was in anyway superficial, and by the time we pulled into our favorite burrito place, the discussion had escalated into a full blown argument.

"Fine," he said finally. "Get your freaking diseased stray dog, just make sure that it's your wage that covers you taking him to the veterinary clinic every week, and that it's you who cleans up after it, when it tears apart and makes a mess in the apartment."

Then, as he was shouting this at me over the roof of our car, I realized that I was going to adopt the chihuahua. Not out of spite or a sense of charity, but because it felt like the right thing to do. Moreover, if he couldn't appreciate or respect that, perhaps we were just not suited to be together, never mind have children.

Later on I therefore called the shelter, and asked what conditions exactly the chihuahua in question (who apparently had already been called Art by one of the shelter staff) had actually been diagnosed with. The girl on the phone then listed gum disease and a scratched cornea that would never heal as Art's only real health problems. Everything else, she said, was just his temperament and aesthetics, hence why they had named him Art.

With my mum swearing by holistic medicine for her own animals, I then started trawling the Internet for homeopathic remedies for these two conditions, as well that is, as rough estimates of how much Art would otherwise be likely to cost me in conventional vet bills.

At first however, what I found just seemed too insane for me to take seriously. You see, everyone knows that the worst thing you can do is let your dog eat chicken bones. Hell, someone in my building had around the same time just raced their own dog to the animal ER, after it had eaten a discarded buffalo wing while out walking.

On the Internet however, there seemed to be a whole host of people in the holistic animal health world, who actually swore by feeding their dogs completely raw joints of meat and pieces of chicken carcasses, specifically so as to keep their pets healthy.

Of course, there are just as many comments underneath such advice deploring the practice.

I was relieved though, to find a few more sober articles praising coconut oil as a great natural antibiotic which can be used safely in both human and animal eyes. This being the case, I started planning to adopt Art on the basis that I might at least be able to treat his eye condition, without having to take biweekly trips to our local veterinary clinic.

A week later then, and with a much more agreeable significant other in tow, I picked Art up from the shelter and brought him into what was then I and Gary's shared apartment in Middle River.

Moreover, although I didn't know it at the time, Art was destined to change my entire outlook on the world.

In fact, it's largely because of him that I have become the woman that have between 2008 and the present.

Of course, it was a rocky road to start with. Art being almost impossible to potty train, was actually the reason that Gary broke up with me later that year.

To clarify however, the reason that I have introduced Art here (who's just turned 14 by the way) is because it was him of all people/canines, who forced me to re-evaluate everything that I then thought that I knew about dieting, not to mention human and animal health and nutrition.

You see, something struck a cord with me when I stumbled upon the debate as to whether or not feed dogs and cats such as Art, species appropriate diets. Or to keep things simple, raw meat, bones and organs, over conventional dog and cat food.

In fact, I was initially fascinated by this debate because it was so simple. On one side there were people who had checked out the ingredients of store bought pet food and were saying, "hey, this stuff is actually really toxic. We've therefore decided to feed our animals human grade quality cuts of meat and guess what? They recover from disease better, live longer, don't have any dental problems and seem in general much happier."

On the other side, there were then just as many people arguing that people who fed their animals raw meat and bones were practically killing them.

Bacteria in the meat was going to make their pet sick at some point, bone fragments were both a choking hazard and had the potential to fatally puncture an animals gut. And aside from all that, standard pet food had been vetted for fifty years by 'experts' in pet health and animal care.

The more however, that I started to research the facts for myself, the more I started to lean towards maybe feeding Art a raw diet. You see, if the pro-raw people were right, it was actually the 80% grain content and abrasiveness of kibble that caused most canine dental and oral health problems in the first place.

Moreover, on researching what actually goes into standard dog and cat food I was mortified.

It is acceptable for example, for euthanized animals such as cats and dogs to be rendered into the kibble, that living cats and dogs then eat themselves everyday.

In fact, in many meat meal rendering plants, euthanized dogs and cats are regularly thrown into rendering vats whilst still inside the plastic body bags that the veterinarian who euthanized them placed them in on the advent of their death.

As if that wasn't bad enough, dead, disabled, disease ridden and dying livestock, deemed unfit for human consumption are also used, and the way that such meat protein is made safe, is via it being heated to extreme temperatures before being spun in a centrifuge to separate the fat from the mixture.

The problem with this process however, is that the heat itself renders healthy fats and protein rancid and toxic. Whilst Sodium Pentobarbital, (the drug used to euthanize peoples pets) itself survives this process and can be measured as still chemically active in pet food in your local store.

Further, to put this in some kind of real perspective for anyone who might struggle to accept that they have been feeding Fido well......Fido, Los Angeles alone, sends 200 tons of cat and dog carcasses to pet food rendering plants each and every month.

Before however, I jumped straight in and started throwing Art whole chicken backs and turkey necks, I researched pet raw feeding in excruciating detail.

Most dogs for example, never learn to actually chew their food. Instead they literally inhale it from their bowls and with this being the case, the last thing that you want to do is throw a chicken leg or a rack of pork ribs their way. Rather, it's best practice to keep hold of such items for what can in some cases be months until their natural chewing reflex starts kicking.

Similarly, I discovered that whilst egg whites are poisonous for dogs, raw egg yolks are along with apple cider vinegar, and secreting organs such as kidneys, are the canine equivalent of super foods.

As it turned out, not only did Art love all of the above, but his own chewing reflex was in top form.

In fact, within a week he was giddily wrestling with chicken drumsticks and pork shank pieces like a pro.

Furthermore, his teeth and gums did start improving. In fact, after six months he was for all intensive purposes a completely different dog. His coat was incredible, most of his teeth were pearly white, his energy levels were fantastic, and despite the fact that he was still covered in scars, he looked beautiful.

Because I had such success treating Art holistically through diet alone, I then ditched the vet we had been using in favor of a 100% holistic practice in Baltimore, and since then we have never looked back.

However, despite the fact that I had by 2009, educated myself enough on dog and cat food, to politely berate anyone in the pet food aisle at my local Safeway, I was still at the same time piling my own shopping cart each week, with chips, diet soda, and processed low calorie ready meals. Not to mention sliced cold meats and specialty breads and candy.

Don't get me wrong, I did think to myself occasionally that it might be worth looking into how processed food for people was manufactured. However, like the majority of American's I simply assumed that there must be some kind of entity of infallible and inarguable reason out there, which made certain that everything that I ate was thoroughly tested and put through stringent series' of quality control tests.

Then in August of that year, someone shared a link with me on Facebook, to an online documentary about one of America's biggest genetic modification companies, and I was floored.

Of course, I knew that I would have to verify each of the specifics, but if what I had watched was genuine, it demonstrated unequivocally that I needed in the very least case, to quickly start rethinking my food purchasing habits.

You see, I knew that genetic modification of America's food was under way. However, when you live like I did then, listening to just MSNBC every day while you have breakfast, and catching shows like The View, to keep you up to date on current events, you really only get one side of the story.

Then, as I set about verifying how our food is genetically modified, as well as reviewing for myself the results of what independent studies had been carried out by then, I started to also look at the amount of additives I was consuming.

I then got brave enough one day to stand naked before my dresser mirror, and I ask myself, "okay Chelsea, are you actually overweight? Or is what you are seeing here the cumulative effect of a lifetime spent slowly poisoning yourself?"

You see, when I thought about it in mind of the amount of crap I was eating in even my low calorie and supposedly nutritionally sound ready meals, I didn't actually look fat. Rather I looked bloated and swollen.

I didn't I then realized, look unhealthy because I was overweight, which is what I had always covered up with make up and told myself was something I could remedy by loosing a few pounds. Rather, I looked overweight because I was unhealthy. And then I felt like kicking myself.

I had after all, for nearly a year by this point, made sure to feed Art only the best of the best. He'd had either sardines and an egg yolk for breakfast or a raw pork chop bone served with a mix of spinach, carrot, sweet potato and lentils.

For dinner, I'd then always made sure to feed him chicken on the bone, or ribs served once in a while with organ meats, and I'd put together this diet with Arts overall health always in mind.

The egg yolks and spinach were great for maintaining healthy eye sight. Including 10% organ meats in his diet, was a great way to make sure that he got the essential vitamins, minerals and digestive enzymes that he needed everyday. And varying between chicken and pork and sometimes turkey, was a great way to keep him enthused about meal times. Not to mention great for maintaining healthy teeth and gums.

I on the other hand, had been feeding myself low fat and low cholesterol chips and sandwich spreads, which every time I ate them, had essentially been stripping me of the vitamins and minerals I needed.

I'd been guzzling zero sugar content soda which perversely is composed in part of chemical molecules, side effects of which include weight gain and diabetes. And I'd been chewing through grilled cheeses every evening, that had a massive Aluminum, Bromine, and Sodium Stearoyl Lactylatepottassium content, not to mention hydrogenated soy and vegetable oil.

In fact, I'd essentially been feeding my dog Art, better than I'd been feeding myself, and despite the fact that I'd watched him visibly get fitter and healthier, it had never until this point crossed my mind that more wholesome food might actually be better for humans also.

I therefore started to cut out things like chips and candy completely. However, as I proceeded to educate myself further, I realized that processed food isn't just chips, candy and ready meals.

I realized by chance for example, that a jar of pickles that I had in the cupboard was listed as containing Sodium Benzoate, a known carcinogen widely used as a commercial preservative. Similarly, despite being advertised as ultimately healthy due to being low fat and sugar free, I found lemon Jelly and cheese crackers at the back of my cupboard, both of which contained Yellow 5, the coal tar derivative we talked about earlier.

I then brought to mind a book that I'd been given comparing the Atkins and the then new and upcoming Paleo diet, and I started to get angry.

You see, whilst Atkins seemed to be fine with allowing artificial sweeteners into your body, the Paleo diet that everyone was raving about, was really just a branch of the wheat and grains are evil crowd. One that although wholesome sounding, didn't mention anything in its advocacy of high fish and meat consumption, in regard to the risks posed by mercury toxicity.

Such musings then made me sit down and think about the diet industry in general. Could it be, I wondered, that somehow the diet industry is all in on it together? That really the people who's books I had read, were really just into making money and as such didn't want to rock the proverbial boat too much?

I mean look at Atkins. What started as a book by a nutritionist in the early 2000's, has since become an industry in of itself. Atkins frozen meals however, are loaded with soy and cornstarch which the company itself has admitted it can't advertise as GMO free....Because they are not.

Likewise, the leading calorie counting regimens out there, themselves support a range of ready meals. However, all of these contain corn and soy derivatives, as well as buckets of chemical emulsifiers, and industrial pesticide ingredients like Disodium Phosphate. (All deemed of course, perfectly safe for human consumption).

Then there is the recipe book business.

After all, once someone buys a book on any given dietary regimen that leaves them a bit flummoxed for meals that they can now put together, they then often go in search of a recipe book to live their life by.

Then there are classes, support groups and memberships that people are encouraged to take out, in order for them to get to meet other people on the same regimen as they are. Then there are gym memberships. And lets not forget the fee of the professional nutritionist, who it is advised that you make an appointment with prior to changing your diet in the first place.

Of course, I'm sure that the diet and health and nutrition industry is topped full of some truly fantastic people. However, in 2009, when I actually started thinking for myself for a change, I realized that America's diet industry itself, is a significant contributor to America's exponentially increasing waistline. Not to mention the nations exponentially deteriorating health.

You see, conflicting sets of do's and don'ts just aren't healthy. Moreover, some regimens openly advocating consumption of things like artificial sweeteners isn't just hypocritical, it's outright dangerous.

I decided to therefore put together my own regimen. One which at first incorporated calorie counting, whilst striving to avoid any and all foods containing chemical additives and traces of GMO.

I quickly realized however, particularly when it came to bread, that I simply couldn't avoid the additives and the aluminum, and the cancer causing coloring agents.

You see, although freshly baked bread in any store you might bring to mind might look wholesome, the dough its all baked from, is still all industrially preprepared.

This being the case, I started baking my own bread. However, as soon as I did that, I lost control completely of being able to count the calories that I was consuming.

In the end then, I simply gave up. What I couldn't allow myself to do however, was risk putting GMO or any kind of additives back into my diet. I mean how was I going to feel about myself in five or ten years time when I might develop some kind of cancer?

I therefore carried on baking my own bread. In fact, I still made and ate everything that I had on my home made diet plan, which was how I got into the habit of cooking up soups and baking every weekend. I was not however, counting calories.

When I then started to loose weight anyway, I almost immediately associated this weight loss with the amount of soup which I had been eating, and sure enough I filled out again when I was eating more protein. By Christmas however, people were starting to congratulate me on how well I looked and ask what I'd done to loose weight, and that's when I started to realize, that actually I had discovered a new way to diet. It just wasn't one that could offer anyone the immediate results that they often wanted.

Moreover, I realized that this weight loss was not something attributable solely to what I was eating.

Rather, I had through increased activity in the kitchen, actually increased my overall physical activity level. Hell, my Saturday baking days are a workout in themselves. More importantly than that however, I had slowly corrected for the better, my own psychological relationship with what I was eating.

As crazy as it therefore sounds, the story of my own weight loss, and return to a state of optimum physical health was instigated initially by my dog, Art.

The point is however, that my improved upon health only came about due to me actively starting to do my own research and this is something that you are going to have to do to.

In fact, in my opinion, reading a book and then starting to try and live your life by the idea that that book's tried to sell you, is one of the worst things that people can do to loose weight.

This book is therefore only meant to be the first stepping stone of your own journey to better dietary health.

Whilst advising people however, on how they can legitimately loose weight and regain their vitality, I'm afraid that it is also necessary to look critically at what other dietary regimens are currently being advocated, and perhaps suggest a few reasons as to why they shouldn't be.

Sinners Dressed As Saints

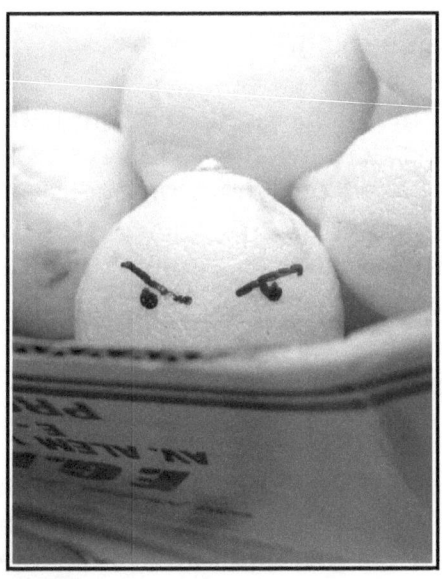

"But isn't it just paleo with bread?" My mum asks me when I tell her that I'm thinking about writing about my regimen. "Don't get me wrong, I think it's a great idea, I just don't want you to be disappointed." [15]

"Besides, it's not actually anything new. You just cook like people used to, and you've happened to

15 Image courtesy of   to Roman Volkov of Romanvolkov.ru

find that it's a great way to loose weight and stay healthy."

"You're right," I say watching Darren, my partner play with my niece Katy, in my mums yard. "Apart from the paleo thing."

And my mum is right. Nothing that I have discovered is actually new. However, although my regimen is based on wholesomeness and common sense, the simple fact of the matter, is that your average American routinely disregards such wholesomeness in favor of convenience.

Further, most people simply aren't aware of how much junk they are putting in their body.

Where Joe America sees a turkey sandwich and a glass of milk, I see azodicarbonamide, a GMO corn and soy fed turkey pumped full of vaccines and antibiotics, and a glass full of cancer causing 1GF-1.

What I want therefore, is a chance to say: "Hey Joe, you're not seriously thinking about putting that in your kids lunch box are you?"

I want to speak to people who are stuck in this emotional conflict cycle, where they feel too fat to go out and meet people and actually enjoy their lives, and so just stay in with only their own anxiety for company. And I want to say "hey, there is a way out of this you know. In fact, how about we start moving together in the kitchen and then see if we can't start going out to catch a movie occasionally?

More than all that though, I want to look out over my own yard one day and see Darren playing with our own kids. Kids who when they go to school, I don't have to worry about the MSG, or the aluminum. and the olestra and the aspartame being served up in the cafeteria every lunch time.

I want a world for my kids that genuinely looks out for their well being, rather than that of the share holders of whoever makes their favorite brand of cheese strings.

Most of all though, I want to grow old free of fully preventable diseases, while watching my kids thrive and bring into the world their own similarly as thriving children.

However, no man or woman is an island, and I can't make America better all by myself. What's the use after all, in working to raise wholesome children, if the world which I'm eventually going to have to leave them in is anything but?

It is my hope then, that I can strike a cord with people. That some people will at least try living and cooking like I'm trying to advocate, and see and feel for themselves the results.

You see, if that happens, a future me might not

have to battle so hard to get my future kids school to serve additive free, possibly even organic school meals.

What I also want to do however, is try and put an end to the faddist and physiologically dangerous way that America presently tries to loose weight, by blindly following whatever dietary regimen is in fashion at any given moment.

Hopefully I have already managed to do this to some degree with calorie counting regimens that encourage purchase of their own low calorie ranges of ready meals. These meals are after all, in some cases so chocked full of additives that at least one brand that I found online recently, had superstitiously omitted to include the ingredients for each of their products.

Don't get me wrong here though. Calorie counting and sticking to one of these agencies diet plans will make you loose weight if you are committed.

The only problem is that you will be saturating your body in chemicals, that although they might not have a noticeable effect immediately, will adversely effect your health in the long term.

Moreover, what I find personally despicable, is the fact that such regimens could blow the lid off the additive, GMO and artificial sweetener market, at any time they wanted. They do after all, have massive amounts of monetary subscribers, as well as the time and resources to pioneer credible research. Not to mention the prerogative.

Here's the kicker though. You're simply no use to these people if you're skinny. They need and want you to be overweight. Hence why America's biggest calorie counting dietary companies are a revolving door. Someone overweight joins, gets their figure back, leaves, gets fatter again, joins again, loses weight again, leaves again, and gets even fatter, etc, etc.

As for Atkins, they are guilty of both additives in ready meals, and ignoring the fact that the quality of meat, fish and dairy, varies hugely depending on how that produce is fed and reared in the first place.

Yes it's great that you can have steak and eggs as often as you like, but don't you want to know whether your eggs have had mercury, antibiotics, and GMO, fed and injected into them?

In fact, in my opinion, Atkins intentionally doesn't draw on the fact that people should only eat organically sourced animal protein, because then the regimen would be impossible for most people to be able to afford to follow.

Less followers would then equal less book sales, not to mention drastically increase the production costs of Atkins own range of ready meals.

Juicing in the meanwhile, is a great way to top up your body nutritionally. (Providing that you're not putting shop bought puddings chocked full of sweeteners in whatever you are juicing). However, it's simply not sustainable for the long term.

As for intermittent fasting, things in that field just get messy. Interpretations of the regimen say that you can eat literally as much of whatever you want, as long as you fast for two days a week.

This however, is just insane. You see, intermittent fasting has been practiced for thousands of years for health and religious reasons, and there is absolutely no question in regard to the practices physiological and psychic benefits.

Come on though America. If you're fasting because you're overweight, you obviously have a poor relationship with food, both emotionally and intellectually.

Emotionally you're probably under the belief that you need to be thin before you can be worth anything, even to yourself. And with this being the case, you likely comfort eat whenever you feel like you will never become the person you want to be.

Intellectually then, you probably don't really know the first thing about nutrition, and therefore don't really understand, that a lot of what you are eating is actually just as deadly as it is fattening.

Sure you know about carbs and calories. However, whenever someone like me comes along and says "hey, you see, that soda that you're drinking? Well do you know that some of the stuff that's in there actually gets metabolized as formaldehyde? You know? The stuff they pump corpses full of to keep them looking fresh?" It's simply too much for you to get your head around.

This being the case, all intermittent fasting does is emotionally reward your comfort eating by saying "hey, here's five full days where you can eat as much as you want!" Before saying "okay, now you have to starve yourself for two days, because you've been bad."

Meanwhile, the regimen doesn't address the fact that the most optimal way to start correcting this poor relationship, is to start being more mindful of what it is that we are actually eating.

Lastly then, there's my pet hates of the wheat is evil crowd, and the let's all just eat like we did 20,000 years ago, paleo diet people.

I mean are you seriously telling me, that wheat having been cultivated for thousands of years has made it worse to consume than aspartame?

Are you really trying to tell me that some Americans abroad not being able to fit on European toilet seats, is down to the bread and pasta that we eat, and not the additive infused sandwich, ice cream, fried chicken, burger, and Mexican grills that we have on every freaking street corner?

You see, Europeans eat bread too. Grains in fact, have been a staple in peoples diets for as long as recorded history. However, it has only been since we started tinkering with our diets chemically and genetically, whilst making it a national past time to go everywhere with a bottle of soda in hand, that obesity and diabetes have ran rampant.

In fact, blaming everything on bread is tantamount to simply blinkering ourselves to the big genetically modified and additive bloated elephant in the room.

Paleo meanwhile, might sound great. But listen kids, before we invented agriculture, your average Joe was far from dining on steak each evening.

Hunting was one of the most dangerous things you could do in the palaeolithic era. We didn't ride horses, we didn't have guns, and all the game that there was, traveled in herds far superior in size to what you might see on National Geographic or today's Discovery Channel.

This being the case, early man has been

archaeologically proven to have for the most part been a scavenger. One who would wait until a kill had been made and devoured by a natural predator, before helping himself when that predator had left, to whatever parts of the carcass were still salvageable.

With predators usually leaving the heads and feet of of their pray, palaeolithic man subsequently dined on brains and eyeballs and cartilage, not tenderized pork loins.

Moreover, when a kill was made by a group of human hunters, it could be tens of kilometers away from their then encampment. This being the case, the women and children often wouldn't eat consecutively from day to day. Really then, the paleo diet should be incorporated with intermittent fasting.

However, what upsets me the most about the paleo and Atkins diets, is the respective regimens promotion of day to day diets high in animal protein.

You see, carotenoids, the natural pigments which give fruit and vegetables their color are proven to be powerful cancer cell combatants.

Working as powerful antioxidants inside our bodies, the more carotenoids in a persons diet, the better protected they are against, cancer, heart disease, and autoimmune disorders.

This being the case, you don't need to be vegetarian to get the benefit, but no diet should advocate eating meat and tubers, over fruit and vegetables.

Moreover, with the paleo diet taking a dim view of dairy, and subsequently being quite dietary restrictive in many regards, it's not really a diet at all. Rather it's a fad just like Atkins was.

Give it a few years and there will be a new regimen doing the rounds, and just like Atkins, most people who jumped on the caveman bandwagon, will have by then fallen off and be looking for someone else to tell them what to eat and how to think.

However, what I have grown to loath much more than such fads themselves, is most American's blind recital of such dietary doctrines.

Last year for example, I was on a flight to Orlando to meet my friend Robyn, and next to me there were two very well suited and obviously very well to do men from Washington.

"I fasted yesterday," one said to the other as if to make out that he was on route to becoming the next Harry Krishna. "It's amazing what a difference it makes, I do it twice a week."

On overhearing this I looked over to the man in question, letting my eyes rest specifically on the perfect dome that was him between his waist and sternum.

"And the best part about it, is I can eat anything when I'm not fasting," he said taking a bite out of a bacon and cheese melt.

"Good luck," I then thought turning my eyes back to my book.

Similarly, whilst researching for this book, I came upon series' of video blogs on youtube, which I truly believe epitomize everything that is wrong with the human race.

In once series, dieters on one of the leading calorie counting regimens, jump giddily around in front of cameras, as they get ready to show you how to make diet soda chicken.

Obviously then, these people are oblivious to the health risks posed by aspartame. However, what troubled me more, was how these you tubers seemed to be immovable in their commitment to using diet soda as a food ingredient; even when almost every comment underneath some such videos, decried the idea as insane due to the associated health risks.

A second series that I then found came from

England, and was a video a day video blog which had already ran for over a year. And to be fair, the young woman videoing herself was sweet, though at times quite emotional as she struggled with some obvious social anxiety issues. However, this woman was on the same calorie counting regimen, and I could see immediately why it was just never going to work for her.

You see, as part of the calorie counting regimen that she was putting herself through, high calorie snacks such as chips, and candy, were still permissible, so long as each serving was categorized as a 'sin' which she was only allowed a certain number of everyday.

This being the case, this woman's kitchen was topped full of absolute junk, that she had meticulously labeled each portion of, in regard to how many 'sins' each one represented.

Moreover, skipping through a whole years worth of videos, I didn't see any noticeable improvement in the way this girl looked.

If however, I could have just sat down with her, and said "okay honey, why don't we go through your kitchen and see what it is you're actually eating?" I can guarantee that in the same year, I could have had this woman not just looking and feeling physically better, but brimming with the confidence that she so obviously wanted.

Then however, there are people like my friend Robyn.

You see, what my friend Robyn does, is go through huge ups and downs in regard to her weight, like she's on some egregious emotional roller-coaster.

However, the worst part about this, is that when something emotionally positive happens in her life, such as her finding a new boyfriend, she immediately convinces herself that her weight isn't a problem.

Hence why when I last visited her, she announced to me that she was in the best shape of her life.

Further, whenever Robyn's in this zone, she becomes exactly like a few people I work with. Ones whom if they have a problem fitting into the clothes they want to, or with them not being able to squeeze easily between the desks in our workplace, cite such problems as what they perceive as discrimination.

The outrage that many overweight Americans voice, when Airlines that they wish to fly with, insist on making them purchase two tickets, is a prime example of this.

You see, aside from falling into dietary fad after dietary fad, and blindly promoting each like it's the best thing in the world, one of the biggest problems with overweight Americans, is that they simply can't accept responsibility for their own shape, size and overall health.

Moreover, the diet industry actively encourages people to distance themselves from such responsibility.

For example, in Gary Taubes book 'Why We Get Fat,' Taubes goes to lengths to explain how our bodies do have an optimum weight regulatory system.

This system however, is ordered chiefly by the hormone insulin. One that over consumption of carbohydrates gradually disrupts and interferes with, and resultantly sees us put on weight.

Like William Davis in 'Wheat Belly,' Taubes subsequently promotes the idea that people should perhaps appropriate blame for their weight on society itself being dependent on cash crops such as cereals and potatoes.

Hold on a just a minute though.

You see, what I don't understand here, is why the carbs are coming under fire first, when monoglycerides, artificial emulsifiers found in everything from paleo nut butter, ice cream, pretty much all baked goods, and almost every kind of breakfast cereal; are themselves known insulin disrupters?

Likewise, aspartame, saccharin, high fructose corn syrup and at least fifty other additives in your average Americans diet, are known to inhibit and disrupt insulin production.

Taube's science is therefore great until he blames carbohydrates alone for America being overweight.

Further, all his book achieves by not addressing the additive issue, is the vilifying once again of the wheat grain, which by being held up for America to blame, exonerates for the meanwhile, America's chemical additive industry.

Of course, anyone who follows Taube's advice and cuts out carbohydrates, will loose weight.

In the long term. However, insulin disrupting monoglycerides will still abound in cheese, yogurt, preprepared soups, and sauces, and a plethora of other things people eat everyday.

This being the case, America, just like she always does, will drop a dress size for the summer... Before moving up three more whilst waiting for the next selectively researched fad to become popular.

Trust me on this one though America, the last thing that you need is the next fad. You loosing weight and becoming the man or woman who you have always wanted to become, is up to you alone. In fact, all the diet industry is doing, is keeping you running round in circles.

Therefore do yourself a favor, and try dropping the bad science and the food is just fuel complexes, that you have had instilled in you.

Then maybe try dropping the extra pounds that you would do anything to be without.

SO MUCH MORE THAN FUEL

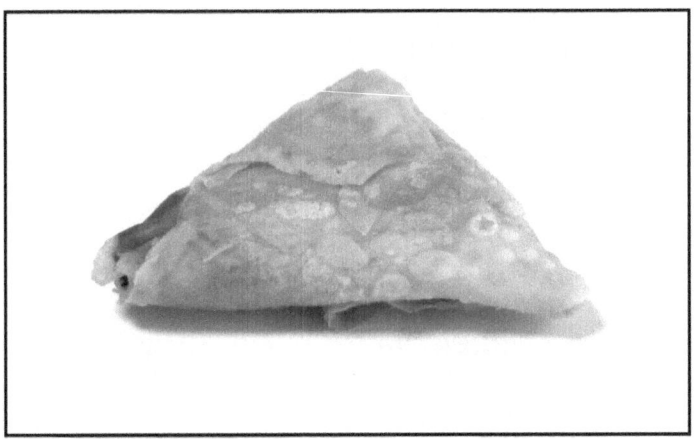

Shortly after my Dad was diagnosed with cancer and we'd circulated the news around our friends and loved ones, my mother got a call from her sister in Baltimore. Her husband Mark, she said, had worked once with a man with prostate cancer. This man however, had apparently survived the disease and had done so by not opting for chemotherapy.[16]

In fact, if Mark remembered right, this man had beat the disease courtesy of a strict dietary regimen.

When however, it was mentioned that the man in

---

16 IMAGE COURTESY OF CONSTANCIA AT WWW.SXC.HU

question was also a vegetarian, my mum and dad politely declined Marks offer to try and find out where his former colleague was now.

Then in 2009, whilst I was running Internet and youtube searches on different food additives and their effects on the human body, I started to stumble upon both written and video testimony of hundreds of people whom had apparently beaten not just cancer, but all kinds of chronic and terminal diseases, through the use of various alternative/dietary derived therapies.

People's children were being diagnosed with autism, only then in some cases, to be fully cured by following strict dietary regimens.

People were being diagnosed with cancer, only then to be able to find that they could manage the condition through diet alone. And people were ditching all sorts of conventional treatments for chronic conditions such as psoriasis, for carefully tailored holistic nutritional regimens. Ones which they said were both cheaper and more effective than conventional medicine.

Moreover, what struck me about these people, was the fact that they weren't trying to sell me or anyone else anything.

Yes, like the raw feeding people whom had already convinced me to feed Art raw, they were advocating a certain theoretical principle. But they weren't actually trying to make me purchase that principle.

They were saying "hey, if your sick with this condition, go down to your store and get this, this and this." And this and this, would usually amount out to be lots of organic colored vegetables and fruits and berries.

Of course, there are some people who do attempt to sell you products of some kind or another. But I'm not talking about these people.

I'm talking about Budwig diet advocates who have solid proof and science behind their way of combating cancer without the need for medication or chemotherapy.

I'm talking about advocates of Gerson therapy. One which has real science behind it, as well as a very real success rate in healing people of not just cancer, but a whole range of diseases.

Johanna Budwig for instance, was a German biochemist and pharmacist, who spent much of her adult life dedicated to researching the importance of essential fatty acids, in regard to human health and vitality.

Discovering during her research, that people with cancer were often deficient in essential fatty acid derived phosphatides and lipoproteins, Dr Budwig

191

subsequently developed a dietary regimen, in which even patients in the advanced stages of cancer, could be reinvigorated and even cured, by consuming a mixture of organic quark or cottage cheese, blended with freshly ground linseeds and cold pressed linseed oil.

Subsequently, thousands of women around the world, have to date cured themselves of estrogen positive breast cancer, even after the disease has metastasized to the bodies bones and vital organs.

Moreover, the Budwig protocol as it is more popularly known, is said by its practitioners to not just thwart terminal cancer, but to also alleviate symptoms of arthritis, as well as work as a preventative of heart infarction.

Of course, American physicians, routinely rubbish the notion that many cancers can in the least case be managed by diet alone. It is not however, the case that this fact isn't backed by nearly a century of clinical research.

You see, Johanna Budwig developed her protocol by building on the 1931 research findings of fellow German Otto Heinrich Warburg, a physiologist who won the then Nobel prize in Physiology and Medicine, for his investigation of the metabolism and respiratory qualities of cancer cells themselves.

In fact, Warburg demonstrated in 1931, that

whereas healthy cells in the human body respire aerobically, (in that they metabolize oxygen) cancer cells thrive in anaerobic conditions. Ones produced in the main, by consumption of glucose.

Indeed, sugar consumption itself, has subsequently been known since 1931, as being a key contributor to people developing cancer in the first place.

Budwig's protocol was therefore designed to oxygenate the bloodstream, and effectively starve cancer cells of the environment which they need to successfully respire, reproduce and metastasize.

Further, far from being a quack or new age pseudo spiritual health practitioner, Budwig herself was nominated no less than six times for the Nobel prize in regard to her work.

What we do therefore, when we think of food merely as fuel for our bodies, is distance ourselves from the fact that what we eat is the principle determinant of our present and future states of physical health.

Yes, we seem to be able to accept that if we eat beans, we will likely develop flatulence. Or that if we drink lots prune juice, we may suffer laxative effects. Similarly, we know that ginger can ease an upset stomach, and it is widely known among neurologists, that high fat and very low carb diets can prevent seizures in epileptics who don't respond to medication.

However, when it comes to informing someone that the Red 3 and Red 40 coloring agents in American condiments, gelatins, baked goods, and confectionery, are known carcinogens. Or that by blending organic quark cheese, crushed linseeds and flaxseed oil, you can mitigate the symptoms and spread of cancer, people just can't bring themselves to accept such matters.

In fact, we don't just rubbish and disregard such information. Rather, when a parent decides against putting their child through chemotherapy, or even against having their child vaccinated, American society aggressively attempts to maintain the status quo, by involving child protective services.

The problem however, is not with those whom break away from the norm and investigate natural ways to mitigate disease.

Rather, America is a society which in truth has always been one based on massive public ignorance.

Founded on the massacre and social and geographical dislocation of America's native inhabitants, we built this country on the back of an appalling slave trade.

Then, even after their emancipation from slavery in

1865, we continued to refuse African Americans the same respect or liberty as white Caucasian Americans, until they had petitioned non-violently for another ninety years.

Rather, while it was imperative for us to realize an idea that was America, we choose to dehumanize the people whom had lived in a sustainable way on the land for centuries before us. Then, when we needed a cost effective work force to build the foundations of the new worlds commerce and industry, we chose to dehumanize people from west Africa, to the point that we put them in manacles and stacked them like sardines, in order to ferry them to work on our cotton and tobacco plantations.

Only emancipating our slaves through a political want to consolidate political power in Washington DC, we then projected a belief that these people were too different and simply not like America's Caucasian population, to ever be deserving of even so much as sharing the same public conveniences with us.

Of course, throughout this ignoble history of ours, we all the while called ourselves Christian and civilized. However, whether we like it or not, the simple fact of the matter, is that for all of our history, America's virtuousness and sense of reason, has always been dictated by what a man or woman in a suit or robe has told us is good for our economy.

Presently then, our national ignorance rests with the idea that the adventures of American science and industry must be at all costs be protected no matter what.

In 2013 for instance, Arkansas, California, Indiana, Nebraska, New Hampshire, New Mexico, North Carolina, Pennsylvania, Tennessee, Vermont and Wyoming, all passed 'Ag-Gag' laws. Ones which make it a criminal offense to publicly publish undercover video taken in any of the aforementioned states factory farms.

Having had profits damaged by footage of live turkey chicks being ground into mincemeat, lame pigs and turkeys rotting alive in atrocious holding pens, and blood being witnessed mixed in with the milk pumped from diseased cows udders, big agriculture business successfully lobbied to have such footages release made a criminal.

This being the case, Americans ignorance in regard to where most of their animal produce comes from, is preserved to the point that organically sourced produce is routinely ridiculed as needlessly expensive, and of no more nutritional worth than regular produce.

In like regard, the GMO industry and big pharma, routinely slurry peoples understanding of the natural world, in order to propagate a perception that products which they produce are far better than those which occur naturally.

Nature is flawed, our scientists tell us. Hence we are duty bound scientifically to better it.

Our chemical and genetic tinkering however, has so far only lead to crops which are nutritionally dead compared to their organic counterparts, and GMO produce which has been shown to cause sterility in second generations of rodents fed it over a full lifetime.

America, is not therefore, better able than nature to organize the world. We are however, bullishly arrogant, and will probably keep on trying to do so, for so long as such is perceived as profitable.

Moreover, this isn't anything new.

In fact, time after time, rather than improve on what nature has already provided for us, we actually interfere adversely with natural produce, just so as to make it marketable.

The leaves and bark of willow trees for example, have been used since 3000BC as a remedy for pain, inflammation and fever. This being the case, salicylic acid, the active component which makes such pain relief possible, has been synthesized by Bayer since 1899, and marketed under the brand name Aspirin.

Common side effects of Aspirin however, ones which include rashes, gastrointestinal ulcerations, abdominal pain, cramping, nausea, and gastritis; are all actually fully avoidable, if one consumes salicylic acid naturally, via chewing willow and myrtle leaves like people did originally.

We need to start to understand therefore, that natural remedies aren't flukes.

Rather, our bodies having spent millions of years consuming wholesome food, have evolved not just to take what they need to grow, but to co-exist in such a way with nature, that or bodies actively utilize compounds in the food that we eat, so as to combat disease.

Fruit, vegetables, herbs, seeds, fish, meat, and even often derided dairy products, are therefore all as powerfully medicinal as they are nutritional.

This being the case, when we belittle foods health giving and restorative powers, all we do is divorce ourselves from our own potential to benefit from such properties.

Scientists admit for example, that caretoids, especially red caretoids, like those found in tomatoes, do play a role in cancer prevention and mitigation. Likewise, as well as garlic and turmeric being natural antibiotics, turmeric has been discovered under laboratory conditions, to itself inhibit cancer cell growth.

When however, anyone attempts to advocate a cancer treatment such as the Gerson therapy, one in which a patient has to consume thirteen portions of freshly prepared organic fruit and vegetable juices each day, America's mainstream medical community decries such regimens as quackery.

This despite the fact that patients whom testify to such therapies successes, include several medical professionals.

Moreover, Gerson therapy should be at least trailed clinically to ascertain as to whether or not it can cure cancer.

After all, since caretoids have been scientifically proved to inhibit cancer growth, a regimen in which someone consumes vast amounts of caretoids in such a manner, is theoretically curative.

In fact, America's medical community refusing to carry out such trials, is to me indicative that they know that such could well prove successful.

You see, if such trials were successful, they could well signal the end of not just America's multi-billion dollar conventional cancer treatment industry, but also American agribusiness.

Alternative therapies such as the Gerson therapy and the Budwig protocol, are after all known not to be as effective, unless exclusively organic produce is used in the preparation of the respective regimens juices and fatty acid mixtures.

Rather however, than this being proof that such protocols are ineffective, it has long been known that pesticides used in conventional agriculture, actually inhibit the caretoids, that are the key health promoting factor in Gerson therapy.

Similarly, with 1GF-1 in non-organic dairy produce being a known cancer promoter, it is plain common sense that one would use organic quark or cottage cheese if following the Budwig protocol.

Whether however, mainstream America likes it or not, nutrition based cancer regimens such as Gerson therapy, have over sixty years of documented success in treating cancer.

That said, I am not making reference here to these protocols in order to convince anyone who might be sick themselves, to choose them over conventional treatment. I know the basics of such regimens, and I have educated myself to the point where if I get sick, I personally will choose such a protocol over conventional medicine. However, I'm not an expert.

If anyone reading this is therefore affected in

anyway by what I'm talking about here, all I can do is advise that you read Charlotte Gersons book, 'Healing The Healthy Way.'

What I am trying to say however, is "step the hell away from the Big Mac America!"

You see, for the most part, our relationship with food at present is simply one in which we get hungry and so we eat. Further, we bring up our children to associate good behavior and birthday celebrations, with candy and trips to our favorite fast food restaurants.

American teenagers in fact, now routinely hang out at their local burger place.

Meanwhile, millions of overweight Americans subsist day to day on dietary regimen endorsed snack foods and ready meals, while millions more spend their waking hours avoiding any kind of carbohydrates, and even more millions run around counting calories, while desperately trying to find a way to calculate whether or not they can have that slice of deep pan pizza that's been on their mind since breakfast.

What every single American seems to have forgotten however, is that food isn't just fuel. Rather, it's the most important thing in our lives and should be treated with the same kind of reverence as we afford money, our smart phones, and all the material things in our lives.

Food keeps us alive and maintains us. We shouldn't therefore, be absent mindedly pouring half and half over bowls of additive infused and artificially colored 'all natural' GMO cereal each morning. Nor should we be unthinkingly throwing MSG and olestra infused chips down our necks at our every convenience.

Rather, we should be getting exited about how much lycopene there is in your average tomato and thinking "hey, I wonder what really thinly sliced tomato would be like for breakfast on a sun dried tomato bread roll with sardines and a drizzle of olive oil?"

We should be stewing steak and cooking pastry tops in the oven, whilst thinking "hey, if I add a couple of bell peppers, grated carrot, and mushrooms just before I turn off the heat, I can preserve all the antioxidants!"

We should be adding a teaspoon of turmeric to our risotto as it gets ready, knowing that this way we get the full benefit of the curcumin. And we should be looking forward to getting home from work, so that we can finally try that Sicilian olive chicken recipe, with those parsnip and sweet potato slices we like roasting with a peppering of curry powder.

Moreover, we should be juicing once a week. Not

because we plan to try and drink ourselves thin, but because we know that doing so is a great way to stay healthy.

Likewise, Rather than getting hung up on what we look like because of how big we are, we should be getting hung up on how unhealthy we are. Then we should be saying to ourselves "hold on, I could stay hung up on this, or I could interpret this as my own personal starting point, for my own personal nutritional adventure."

You see, I don't want you to feel like you can't have your favorite brand of cookies because they might go straight to your hips. I want you to not want those cookies any more anyway, because of the additives, flavorings and colorings that you have educated yourself enough about, to know that you don't want them in your body.

Then I want you to still be able to enjoy yourself, by making your own cookies using organic honey and molasses instead of refined sugar.

Further, when someone then asks why you have decided to do all your own cooking and baking, I want you to say something like: "Well I found out that whereas in the 60's your average American ate about a kilogram of chemical additives every year, we now each consume over five kilograms, and this increase correlates exactly with increases in chronic disease and obesity. - As such I've decided to educate myself on health and nutrition, and add a few years back to my life, rather than put any more extra pounds on my backside."

You see, it's really very simple. There are books and tapes and classes and therapists out there, who all promise that they can stop you overeating by making you confront why you overeat psychologically.

People do not however, overeat on home made turkey casserole and goulash served with home made garlic bread rolls. They overeat on fast food, snacks, preprepared meals and confectionery.

Further, although you may indeed have genuine issues with your childhood and upbringing that drive you to over indulge when it comes to chips and wedges of chocolate cake, our instinct for survival and self preservation completely overrides these.

Instead therefore, of trying to program people to eat less, the best thing that anyone can do is educate themselves on what's in their food, so that their sense of self preservation can kick in and say, "er, Chelsea? You do know that we can't eat any of this garbage don't you?"

Better still, if you're a parent, take a moment to start looking at what your kids are eating, and see if you don't start quickly feeling violently outraged.

Did you know for example, that dimethylpolysiloxane, an industrial adhesive and defoaming agent, is actually added to most of the fryer oils of your kids favorite burger and fries restaurants?

When therefore, your teenagers are hanging out at their favorite burger place, or you're taking your younger kids to their favorite fast food place as a treat after school, keep in mind that all these future happy memories of theirs, all come with the price tag attached of you having paid for them to eat window putty.

Besides, wouldn't it be nice to all eat together again properly?

~ It's Not The Freaking Wheat America ~

BAD SCIENCE? REALLY?

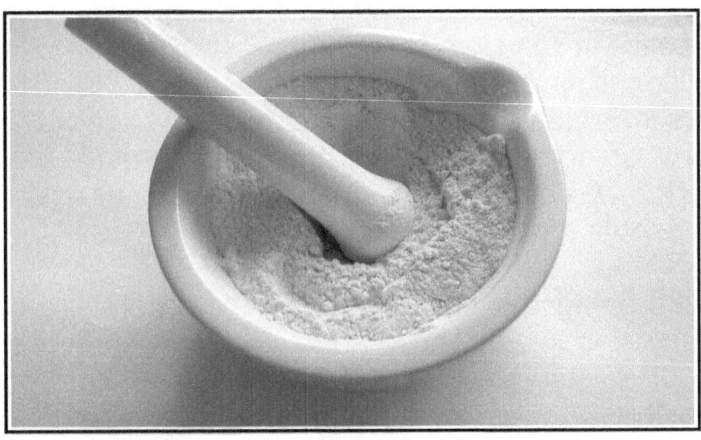

"Let's say that you weren't as lucky as you are," Kevin O'Leary of Canada's CBC current events show, The Lang and O'Leary Exchange, says to fourteen year old Rachel Parent.[17]

"Let's say you were born in an Asian country, you're fourteen years old, your only food is rice that has no vitamin A in it, you're going blind and then you die. Five hundred and fifty thousand people your age die that way every year."

"Alternatively," he continues. "A company like Monsanto could come along and offer you a

17 IMAGE COURTESY OF POTTASCHE AT WWW.SXC.HU

genetically modified form of rice which includes vitamin A, that can save your eyesight and your life. How do you feel about that Rachel?"

In the debate being referenced here, Kevin O'Leary, a man who is worth approximately $300 million, then stated as the fourteen year old girl he was interviewing affirmed that she was against any form of genetic modification of food, that such a notion was essentially a death sentence for millions of people around the world.

This being the case, the idea that there are too many people on the planet, and that genetically modification of staple food crops is the only feasible way to combat famine and malnutrition, was once more propagated in defense of America's leading agribusinesses.

Moreover, this supposition was coupled, as is often the case, with the suggestion that anyone therefore against GMO, is equivocal to a dangerous radical. One who's views if they were embraced by society, would lead to the needless death of millions.

Every such thing said in defense of America's genetically modified crop producers, is however, nothing more than deluded, non-factually supported corporate and political fantasy.

You see, in 2008, the United Nations very own Food and Agriculture Organization, announced that it would take only $30 billion of investment from wealthy countries to eradicate world hunger forever.

World hunger had actually increased since 1980, the same report said, directly due to a 58% drop in such investment.

Without however, throwing too many numbers around, the case at present is that if she so wished, the Queen of England could personally end all world hunger, simply by investing some of her personal fortune into agricultural projects in some of the worlds poorest places.

As could any number of American billionaires you might bring to mind.

The idea then, that only genetically modified food can save the world from famine is false.

Further, rather than maligning those whom demand further testing and labeling of such products as anti-science social deviants, we should really be maligning a federal government which spends more in American tax dollars promoting this industry overseas, than it would actually cost to end world hunger forever, in just the space of a single year.

Moving on however, it is not just advocates of GMO labeling, who are purposefully maligned by protectors of American corporatism.

Rather, it is also the case that any whom promote alternative medical therapies such as those discussed in the previous chapter, are routinely denounced as dangerous charlatans. Crooks and con-men out to pray upon peoples physical and emotional vulnerabilities in their darkest hours of need.

At sciencebasedmedicine.org for example, there is a stinging critical analysis of the aforementioned Gerson therapy. One which like many others, attempts to imply that supporters of the protocol are actually on a par with creationists, due their seeming belief that the human body is capable of healing itself, providing that it can be equipped with compounds that nature has provided for it in our food.

Rather however, than imply that human physiology and the ordering of the natural world around us, is indicative of intelligent design of some sort, all Gerson therapy demonstrates, is that the human body can take what it needs from nature, just a little more efficiently than we have ever previously appreciated.

It is an indisputable fact that our bodies depend on being able to acquire nine essential amino acids from the food which we eat, just to survive. Why is it therefore so implausible to assume, that in the same evolutionary time which our bodies have learned to source some of the essential proteins that we need from nature, we could not also have learned to source and utilize the fatty acids and caretoids that we need to help us overcome disease?

Further, accusing promoters of such therapies as soulless profiteers, just doesn't make sense.

If someone wishes to follow such a protocol, they do not need to give their health insurance details to anyone. Nor do they need to purchase any special drugs from people like Pfizer. They can simply start following the regimen, freely in their own time, in their own living space.

Of course, I don't know from personal experience if such will work. However, when I decided to take the plunge and feed my dog Art, a raw diet of meaty chicken bones and organs, I had to overcome the same kind of fear that practitioners of these therapies must go through, when they make personal decisions to go against conventional wisdom.

"OMG! Get that dog to a vet now!" someone posted in a forum in reply to my account of feeding Art raw for the first time. "Everyone knows that you don't give dogs chicken bones, especially not a chi!"

In fact, if it wasn't for Art having lived on the

streets for all of his life, I don't really know if I would have actually done it.

To me though, it was just insane to think that he wouldn't have eaten bones when he was a stray, and so I felt more comfortable with the idea of me feeding him them myself.

Further, Art's teeth firmed up, his gums healed, and he became visibly much healthier, just like the raw feeding people who I hadn't paid a penny said that he would.

Since then in fact, I haven't paid our veterinarian a cent. Aside that is, for what we pay for six monthly check ups.

Indeed, although Art has pretty much reached the end of his natural life span, he really doesn't show the slightest sign of slowing down. Not yet anyway.

This being the case, when I see opinion pieces on GMO, scientific derisions of alternative/nutritional medicine, veterinary experts calling people out for not feeding their pets industry approved kibble, and food industry experts sending in lawyers to deal with anyone decrying the use of chemical additives in our food, I just see a corporate machine that is itself terrified of being called out as criminal.

You see, as far as I'm concerned, I'm not anti-science for saying to people that I believe that GMO should be tested more. Nor am I some kind of snake oil saleswoman, simply for saying "hey, have you heard about holistic medicine and animal care?" And I am certainly not some kind of anti-capitalist activist, simply for saying that really it should be common sense to steer clear of food additives.

Rather, anyone true to the principals of real science would test GMO more comprehensively.

Likewise, if alternative disease and cancer therapies are really dangerous and ineffective, this should be established resolutely in clinical trials. This way if such treatments were found to be without merit, the fact could be published and peoples lives could be saved.

Moreover, as for it possibly not being commonsensical for me to advise people to steer clear of food additives, okay, get rid of the doublespeak lawyers, get some independent scientists in here for a moment, and please, explain to me why substances banned in other countries, not to mention others which have been proven to cause cancer in lab animals, are permissible in America's food supply?

Of course, I don't blame the doctor, the vet or the low level agribusiness employees, for the state that America's presently in. Nor for that matter, do I even blame the lawyers.

You see, when aspiring physicians go to college in America today, nutrition simply isn't something that they focus their study on.

In fact, food courts in America's leading medical universities are populated by McDonald's restaurants, Chick-fil-A's, and grills, and pizza stations.

Even therefore, our next generations of doctors and dietary specialists, are people imbued from the beginning, with the idea that it either doesn't matter what we eat, or that everything is good in moderation.

Similarly, it is leading pet food brands which actually sponsor the diet and nutrition classes at veterinary universities.

In fact, pet food industry representatives actually give guest lectures and present seminars to such budding veterinary professionals.

Similarly, many future veterinarians subsequently sign contracts with such companies, in order to exclusively endorse their products in their own surgeries when they have them.

Likewise, for the men on the ground in America's major agribusinesses, everyday is just another dollar.

Further, when lawyers are assigned cases concerning America's food industry, they can only argue such cases, once they have a medical professional or two on board.

But hey, guess what? These independent medical experts are people who by and large didn't major in nutrition. In fact, if they graduated at any time over the past twenty years, they probably did so from a Med school, where they spent most lunch times, themselves tucking into anti-biotic infused meats and a plethora of flavor enhancers and other additives.

All this being the case, please therefore snap out of this idea that everything is A-okay as long as it is expert or celebrity endorsed.

Earlier in this book for example, I said gee, wouldn't it be great if someone like Angelina Jolie would take a stand against sodium nitrate? You will never however, see any major celebrity endorsing such a campaign. Why? Because quite simply they would find it very hard to find work after.

I mean can you imagine what would happen if a movie star took a stand against GMO corn? You see, yeah, their latest movie might have grossed a few tens of millions of dollars, but I'll bet that's nothing compared to how much money cinemas in the United States make in popcorn sales per annum.

 The only person therefore, who you should trust to make dietary decisions on you behalf is you.

 This being the case, once you have read this book, you should go out there and see for yourself if I'm telling the truth about the olestra in the chips in your cupboard.

 You should go find for yourself, sets of obesity statistics for Americans for the past half a century, and then compare these for yourself, to things like increases in the amount of additives in our food.

 Moreover, when you come across articles and publications on your way, which attempt to vilify naysayers of GMO and alternative medicine, you need to strip such publications down to the bare facts and compare them for yourself, to articles written which promote discussion about such topics. Then it's your job to decide which one is more balanced.

 Most importantly however, you need to start turning over products before you put them in your shopping cart. Then you need to decide for yourself, whether or not you want to change your lifestyle, slowly loose that extra weight that's been getting you down for so long, and start feeling great about yourself.

 You see, avoiding GMO's, additives, hormones, and artificial sweeteners in your diet, by cooking all your own food, will set you on course for long term sustainable weight loss.

You will notice significant improvements in your health and your sense of personal vitality. Further, when you start feeling a closer, more personal bond with your food, you will likely start feeling a stronger bond starting to develop between you and your loved ones.

I can not however, make such a regimen sound as convenient as the one described in the last diet book you read. Neither can I say that you will drop a jean or a dress size in this or that amount of time.

The case is simply that food has become something of a passion of mine over the past seven years. And this has been my most recent attempt to date, to share that passion with other people.

Moreover, although I've said throughout this work that I can't make you thin overnight, here's something that I've noticed over the course of the past seven years:

You see, between 2009 and 2012, I lost nearly one hundred pounds. The truth is though, that I started feeling better about myself almost straight away.

Indeed, in many ways my life got more exciting, and although I haven't really been able to include the social side of this adventure here, you do find when you start the kind of lifestyle that I have, that you start to register as quirky and interesting on other peoples life radars.

This being the case, you start to attract quirky and interesting people into your own life and quirky and interesting things start to happen to you.

In the meantime however, I've watched people like my friend Robyn, who I have repeatedly tried to advise on how to loose weight and get healthy, run round trying every kind of diet that they can. Why? Because they want the immediate results that the latest book they saw featured on Dr Oz promises.

Hence, while I've been starting out on an adventure, in which I've been able to meet some truly incredible people, fall in love, and develop intellectually, politically, and therapeutically within myself; people like my friend Robyn have actually just got bigger and unhappier.

Them chasing unattainable and unmaintainable immediate solutions to their weight, just saw them crash and burn every six months or so just like I used too.

In fact, the seven years that they have spent with many of their lives on hold, trying to find some quick fix for the way that they look and feel about themselves, has by and large been wasted.

Yes, my friend Robyn found a new man, and is presently feeling great about herself. But after a lifetime of friendship, you do start to be able to see though the people that you love's ups and downs to a certain degree.

The question is therefore, where were you in 2009, in regard to where you are right now? Are you bigger or smaller? Has dieting actually ever worked for you previously? Or have you only ever actually lost weight intermittently, before getting tired of a particular regimen and putting it all back on again?

More importantly though, where do you want to be in another seven years? Still living like a dietary yoyo? Or thinking, gee am I glad I decided to put my weight problem behind me the healthy way?

Because hopefully to a few of you, this will be the moment that you will be looking back on.

~ It's Not The Freaking Wheat America ~

GOOD HOUSE KEEPING

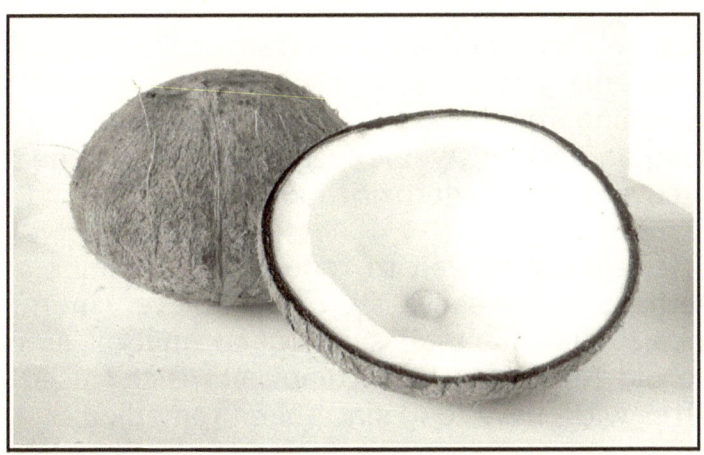

"I just hold it in my mouth for twenty minutes?" Darren asks me looking uncertain. He used to look at me a lot like this when we first started dating. Like every now and then he's not actually talking to me face to face, but through some kind of interstellar Skye video window, showing me as on a completely different planet to him.[18]

"Yes, and then spit it into the toilet but not the sink. And make sure that you don't swallow."

Art looks up from his bed under our front window

---

18 IMAGE COURTESY OF 4FUN AT WWW.SXC.HU

as if in sympathy with Darren. He was after all, the first person/canine that I ever subjected to one of my coconut oil home remedies.

Rather however, than Darren suffering with his eyes, he's had toothache for the past few days and so I'm trying to encourage him to start oil pulling. Oil pulling, for those not familiar with the practice, being an ancient Ayurvedic remedy for oral health and overall bodily detoxification.

Scientifically proven to reduce germ numbers in teeth, gums and saliva, I've oil pulled every morning since 2010 with a table spoon of coconut oil, and all the old teeth and gum complaints that I used to suffer with, have long since been remedied by the procedure.

"And is this going to be immediate? Or is it one of these slow cures of yours?"

"Slow," I say. "But in a week you should already be feeling better. If not it's the dentist I'm afraid."

Rather however, than take you on a tour of a morning in our apartment, I'd like to introduce oil pulling here, as one of the things which you can do if you do change your diet like I've tried to advocate thus far.

You see, you can't magically make your body all better, especially if you have unwittingly put it through a lifetime of dietary abuse like most people who are overweight have.

You can however, do some fantastic things to expedite your return to health.

If you get into the habit of oil pulling for example, you won't just be bettering your own oral health. Rather, thousand's of people attribute oil pulling as being a powerful tool to better digestive health, better skin, better liver and kidney function, and even better eyesight.

It is important though, to use only organic cold pressed oil, preferably sesame seed or coconut.

Personally I like to use coconut as I always have a jar around.

In fact, remember what I said about some vitamins and minerals being fat soluble and subsequently only passing through our gut once they have been picked up by whatever fat you have consumed? Well studies have shown that coconut oil is not just superior to other fats in this respect, but using it regularly as a supplement can even better your bodies processing of caretoids and essential plant enzymes.

As if that wasn't great enough, organic cold pressed coconut oil, can also be used as a natural sun screen. (Having a sun protection factor of 15 it's great for anyone particularly worried about premature aging).

This being the case, both me and Darren use it as a body moisturizer however, because it can be quite greasy, it's worth applying it immediately after showering. Don't ask me why, we've just found that it absorbs better.

Of course, when I decided to start afresh with my diet and health regimen, I didn't try to detox just by oil pulling. Neither though, did I follow a standard detox regimen.

You see, if you're switching from an average American diet to any kind of new one, it is important to detox, primarily so that your body is primed to be able to start absorbing all the new nutrients which you are about to fill it with.

Past detoxing experiences however, hadn't actually left me feeling detoxified.

Sure, some people make out that they feel incredible after spending a week eating a diet rich in green vegetables, onions garlic and beets. Me though, my body just didn't ever seem to respond, and as such I decided to do a full sea salt bowel cleanse to kick start my better health drive.

Having possible adverse medical repercussions, (especially for anyone in poor digestive health) this is however, something that I must insist that you do not attempt to replicate until you have spoken to either your own doctor, or a professional holistic health expert.

Having irritable bowl syndrome at the time, I myself took such advice but had to make a repeat visit to my health practitioner, simply because she herself wasn't actually aware what a sea salt bowel cleanse actually was; and subsequently had to research the matter herself before advising me on it.

First popularized (I think) in the Master Cleanse by Tom Woloshyn, a sea salt flush as it is also called, is where you mix 2-3 teaspoons of unrefined, bleach and additive free sea salt, to a quart of warm water, drink this mixture, and then lie on your right side in the fetal position for twenty to twenty five minutes.

At this point, most people will then get the urge to go to the bathroom and, will (from my own experience) probably go through a succession of 7 to 15 bowel movements.

In many respects in fact, flushing your system in this way is like putting yourself through a kind of internal enema. Moreover, many medical professionals say that the gut shouldn't actually be flushed in this way, because one, it strips us of vital digestive bacteria, and two, our gut and bowels have their own way of cleaning themselves naturally.

For me however, I was concerned that because I had been such a big corn lover previously, I might have bacteria in my gut which had been interfered with by GMO BT toxin. I therefore flushed for three days consecutively, and every day after my final bowel movement, I would make a quick berry smoothie with loads of organic yogurt and kefir.

Meanwhile, rather than juice, I was having incredibly rich vegetable soups each evening, as well as tons of green tea with lemon and grated ginger.

My week of detoxing was therefore composed of three days of salt flushing every morning, organic berry smoothies after each final bowel movement, thick vegetable soups for dinner each evening, (so as to replenish my stock of digestive enzymes) and for breakfast on the fourth through to seventh days, I'd have the berry smoothies that I had originally been having after my bowel cleanses.

(On days one through three, I didn't have anything to eat until my after final bowel movement).

Further, rather than embrace any kind of mindset which sees me detox like this every six months or so, I have ever since then simply continued to drink green tea and lemon as my main beverage throughout each and every day, and just eat as healthy as possible.

You see, you can cleanse your bowel and even your liver as much as you like. However, you can't purge your body of the toxins which it has squirreled away in your fat cells, or for that matter, all the other tissues throughout your body. Not in the same kind of immediate fashion anyway.

Moreover, these toxins are there. When for example, someone does the Gerson therapy, they go through a series of crippling healing responses, in which after a length of time following the Gerson dietary regimen, their bodies wake up to the fact that they are full of toxins and try getting rid of these all at once.

Similarly, after six months of feeding Art raw, he suddenly started to stink and spiral down hill health wise. Luckily however, I'd by that time been chatting regularly with some other raw feeding people in a dedicated Chihuahua forum.

"Don't worry," they said. "This his just Arts body realizing that now is a great time to detox. It might last for up to a month."

This being the case, it is possible to fully detoxifying your body. However, this detoxification is in your case going to take the form of you slowly starting to loose weight.

You see, as you start putting better quality food into your body and are forced to eat in rather than out all the time, your body will start saying, "hey, since there's been no garbage coming through here for a while, maybe we should start trying to clear out some of that ammonium sulfate and polysorbate 60 we've had locked up in those dimples on Lisa here's ass for the past three years."

Do yourself a favor though, and don't think about your initial week priming yourself, or your starting out being more conscious about what you eat, as any kind of actual detoxification program.

Rather, try to start thinking of your body as somewhere where you live. A house, a car, a boat or whatever. Consider then that it's your job to keep it in great running condition and that with this being the case, you're just starting to practice good housekeeping.

You see, detoxing sounds and impresses upon us psychically as medical and in many regards, kind of alarming.

Rather then, than worry about what kind of state your body might be in right now, try and see you planning better stewardship of it, as cause for a celebration of some sort.

In fact it was with such an idea in mind that I

personally decided to ditch coffee when I started this regimen, and decided instead just drink green tea infused with lemon. You see, the lemon not only alkalizes your body making it better oxygenated and healthier, but it also works to de-calcify our joints, arteries and lymph nodes. Whilst green tea in itself is a great antioxidant.

I also decided early on, to be much more selective about even the salt that I season and cook my food with.

Standard store bought refined salt is by and large chlorinated and for all intensive purposes toxic. Sea salt however, isn't refined and is largely toxin free. Better still, some organic shops sell five kilogram bags of pink Himalayan sea salt, mined from the remains of pristine prehistoric seas.

Further, getting in the habit of moving more is also important, but not as you might first assume, solely for the obvious reason of burning calories. Rather, the more you move, the more you encourage circulation of water around your lymph node system itself.

In my case getting Art was a great way to get me moving. Needing to be walked three times a day, I had to drop feeling self conscious about the way I looked just after getting out of bed every morning and just get on with it.

If therefore, one of the things that has so far held you back from joining an exercise class or even just walking around the block everyday, is you feeling too self conscious about yourself, think about getting a small dog.

They make great companions, walking your dog is a great way to strike up conversation with strangers and meet new people, and having something to care about that isn't your job, or what people do or do not think of you, is a great curative of many peoples anxiety problems.

Of course, I'm not saying that you need to get a dog, I'm just saying that in my case it helped a lot.

Lastly, do yourself a favor and ditch the microwave. I'm not sure of the science behind it, but I read somewhere a while ago that plants watered with microwaved water simply don't grow all that well.

This isn't however, the reason that I got rid of mine.

Rather, the age of the ready meal and food convenience, has been greatly aided by peoples adoption of microwave cooking. Then, when I started cooking for myself, my sister gave me a great recipe book for microwave cooking that covered pretty much everything.

Pork loin, baked potatoes, potato chips, meatloaf, lasagna, everything that I wanted to cook and eat for myself, even cakes and peanut butter cups, I could all prepare with next to no effort in the microwave.

I quickly realized however, that this wasn't for me.

By cooking in the microwave, I wasn't after all, actually learning how to prepare the food that I was making. And I missed the actual physical activity of pot roasting bacon pieces and attempting to transform them seamlessly into a mouthwatering carbonara sauce.

Likewise, I missed monitoring quiches that I had in the oven, wanting to make sure that they didn't burn, but also needing to wait for them to firm up before I risked turning the heat down.

A big part of my new dietary experience, was in essence my being in the kitchen and my cooking traditionally.

However, even when I decided to stop using my microwave, it still made me cheat. Rather than start again if I burnt a sauce, I'd ladle what I could save into a microwave dish and finish it in there.

Similarly, if I got home late and couldn't be bothered to put the oven on to reheat some lasagna that I had preprepared, whilst cooking up a side of vegetables, I'd simply throw two portions of lasagna in the microwave.

Hence I actually started overeating for a small while, due simply to settling for the convenience of the microwave over even the tiniest effort it would have taken me to eat a little bit healthier.

Realizing therefore, that I risked falling into a new kind of negative cycle with my diet, I simply decided to get rid of my microwave altogether.

Moreover, I'd strongly recommend that you do too. In the very least case you will be saving on your power bills.

GOODNIGHT AND GOOD LUCK AMERICA

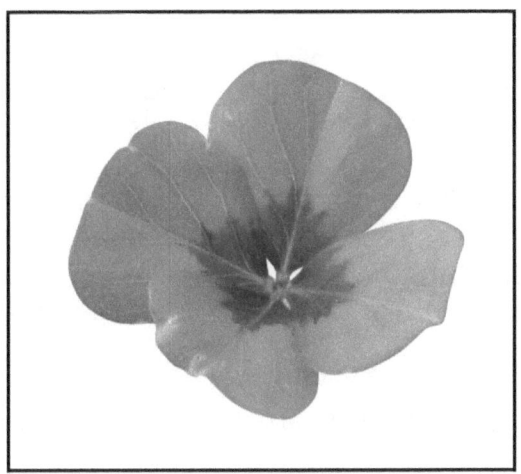

When I started this book, I didn't really realize how much of myself I would actually put into it.[19]

I have not however, shared my own experience in changing my diet and lifestyle, in order for anyone to try to emulate it entirely.

If you're a smoker like I am/used to be, don't run out there now and buy a carton and think that it's okay, as long as you only do so once every six

---

19 IMAGE COURTESY OF NIELS TIMMER AT WWW.VORMSPEL.NL

months. That's my coping strategy not yours.

Please however, do start to seriously think about regaining your health and vitality, by cutting out everything artificial in your diet.

Moreover, please don't close this book and try and convince yourself that I have exaggerated, either the known effects of many food additives, or the pervasiveness of them in America's food chain.

You see, additives are hugely detrimental to your health, and they really are everywhere. Even canned food and drinks (as consequence of the canning process itself) are carriers of the epoxy derivative bisphenol-A.

(As for that matter, are many brands of bottled water).

Further, part of the problem at present, is that when people see Yellow 5, or partially hydrogenated vegetable oil listed in the ingredients table of their favorite chips, they think for some reason, that these ingredients represent some kind of naturally sourced coloring and emulsification compounds.

In fact, the last thing that people will likely associate with such ingredients, is giant high pressure cooking vats, in which catalysts like nickel are introduced to purposefully transform naturally occurring fats, into something that's just one molecule away from being plastic.

Nor will people seriously consider for any length of time, that the caramel or yellow color of their bread, pasta, or candy, is actually attributable to coal tar.

Further, I've just mentioned a tiny number of additives. The case is however, that there are over 6000 industrial chemicals in the average American diet, none of which occur naturally in food, and none of which your body has the faintest idea how to safely process.

In fact, I can't tell you which one it is, (due simply to the fact that I'd likely be sued quite quickly) but the following is a list of ingredients for just the bun of one of America's leading burger chains:

Enriched Flour (niacin, iron, thiamine mononitrate, riboflavin, and folic acid), Water,
Sugar (sucrose or high fructose corn syrup),
Sesame seeds,
Vegetable shortening,
Salt,
Wheat gluten,
Yeast,
Yeast Food (calcium sulfate, potassium iodate, and/or ammonium sulfate),
Dough Conditioners (polysorbate 60, calcium peroxide [oxidant], calcium salts, sulfates,

phosphates, and ammonium salts),
Dough Strengtheners (sodium and/or calcium-2-steroyllactylate or ethoxylated ono- and diglycerides),
Dough Softeners (mono- and diglycerides, and/or protease enzyme), mold inhibitor (calcium propionate),
Preservative (potassium sorbate),
Oxidation/Reduction additives (ascorbic acid, potassium/calcium iodate, alpha-amylase, azodicarbonamide),
Leavening Agent (monocalcium phosphate).

Further, you might be surprised to find that many of the specialty breads available in many public supermarkets, are composed of exactly the same ingredients.

What we have presently come to then, is a juncture in America's history, in which to make our bread look better and cost less to produce, we have unaccountable corporatists putting up to twenty different non-naturally occurring ingredients, into one of the very staples of the average American diet.

At the same time though, the people who eat this crap simply don't seem to care.

Either Americans don't know what their food really contains, or they automatically trust the agencies which provide it for them. A feat often accomplished by the use of bright colored packaging, and duplicity stamped on slogans which advertise whatever you are about to eat as 100% natural.

Here's the kicker though kids, I could put sulfur hexafluoride in your buffalo wings and still call them 100% natural. After all, the gas in question is produced by 100% natural volcanic eruptions.

In fact, for a final exemplification of the matter, imagine that you go to a friends house for dinner, where there is a big pot of something simmering away in the kitchen.

As however, you go to see if you can lend a hand, you come across your host putting twenty different drops of twenty different chemicals into what he or she is cooking. Drops which you can visibly see being decanted from vials labeled as Calcium-2-Steroyllactylate, Azodicarbonamide, and Butylated Hydroxyanisole.

Now, would you still feel as comfortable about sitting down to have dinner later?

As it is however, every week I see women who look like Victoria's Secrets worst nightmare, accompanied by intellectually abandoned looking husbands and kids, filling shopping carts with microwavable sausages and pancakes, kids cuisine supposedly healthy ready meals, and fat free potato chips, chock full of such chemicals, and I despair.

You see, we have a really big problem here America.

We're fat, we're ugly and we're getting real sick. And I'm sick of seeing people I know, start reaching for false solutions to this problem, in the form of books that tell them to eat like cave people.

Yes, you need to eat less and yes you need to exercise. But come on, start checking out what you're freaking eating too America!

Moreover, this isn't just about us. This is about the food culture and the eating habits that we are right now imbuing our children with. I mean is it any wonder that we're pumping them full of Ritalin, sending them to fat camp, and seeing a whole generation grow up intellectually dislocated from what real food is?

Of course, my saying such things, usually just leads to people saying: "Err? Chelsea? You do know that everything is all right in moderation right?"

In fact, I've lost count of the amount of people who have went out of their way over the years, to make this specific remark.

There is however, an astronomical difference in me

indulging in home made chocolate fudge cake every couple of weeks, and the rest of America tucking into aluminum. sulfate infused chocolate chip muffins in their favorite coffee shop every afternoon.

You see, this book hasn't been about scaring anyone or insulting anyone. And I say that because I know that there will be people reading this, who see their stopping off in their favorite coffee shop every afternoon, as some kind of wholesome lifestyle choice that they have made.

Rather, I just wanted to try and help people, just like all the other diet books out there say that they want to, and the simple fact of the matter, is that cooking all your own food, and using as many wholesome ingredients as you can, will lead to long term sustainable weight loss. Really, it's that simple.

The only difference between this and most other publications presently on the market, is that I haven't tried to shy away from the real reason why America's health and vitality has been in terminal decline for the past two decades.

I will hope in the very least case then, that I've at least planted a bug in a few peoples ears.

Goodnight then America, and good luck getting to be whoever it is you want to be.

However it is that you try and get there though, please don't just blame wheat for everything.

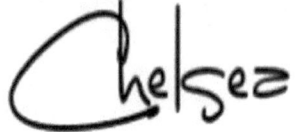

END